Medicinal Perennials
to Know and Grow

MEDICINAL PERENNIALS
TO KNOW AND GROW

DAN JASON *and* **RUPERT ADAMS**

watercolour illustrations by **LYN ALICE**

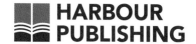

HARBOUR PUBLISHING CO. LTD.
P.O. Box 219, Madeira Park, BC, VON 2HO
www.harbourpublishing.com

ALL ILLUSTRATIONS by Lyn Alice
COVER AND TEXT DESIGN by Libris Simas Ferraz / Onça Publishing
PRINTED AND BOUND in South Korea

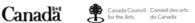 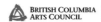

HARBOUR PUBLISHING acknowledges the support of the Canada Council for the Arts, the Government of Canada and the Province of British Columbia through the BC Arts Council.

LIBRARY AND ARCHIVES CANADA CATALOGUING IN PUBLICATION
Title: Medicinal perennials to know and grow / Dan Jason and Rupert Adams ; watercolour illustrations by Lyn Alice.
Names: Jason, Dan, author. | Adams, Rupert, author. | Alice, Lyn, 1958- illustrator.
Description: Includes bibliographical references.
Identifiers: Canadiana (print) 20230213715 | Canadiana (ebook) 20230213774 | ISBN 9781990776465 (softcover) | ISBN 9781990776472 (EPUB)
Subjects: LCSH: Herbs—Therapeutic use. | LCSH: Medicinal plants.
Classification: LCC RM666.H33 J37 2023 | DDC 615.3/21—dc23

Contents

Note

The content of this book is for informational purposes only and is not intended to diagnose, treat, cure or prevent any condition or disease. Plants have distinct effects on different people. It is vital that you consult your health care provider before considering any self-directed treatment of a medical condition, including the use of medicinal plants. Be vigilant when consuming medicinal plants: if you notice any negative effects, discontinue use and consult your health care provider immediately. Some beneficial plants closely resemble other plants that are toxic to humans. Before you consume any plant, consult with an expert to be certain that you have correctly identified it.

Introduction

There are some great reasons to consider knowing and growing the medicinal perennials in this book.

1. They can support your well-being and heal what ails you.
2. They have extremely long histories of safe use.
3. They are all easy to grow and wonderful to observe.
4. They become larger, more beautiful and easier to maintain with every passing year.
5. They are amazing at encouraging biological diversity.

In terms of supporting health and healing what ails you, you're likely to connect with some herbs in this book and not others. But, as a gardener, you might embrace all of them! Revered around the globe as healing medicine for thousands of years, they bring powerful energy to any garden. The medicinal herbs in this book can energize or calm you, stimulate your immune system, give you a good night's sleep, aid digestion, help heal wounds and injuries, tone your organs, change your blood pressure, reverse inflammation and soothe a sore throat.

And they can make you happy!

They have a different kind of beauty and grace than commonly grown food crops. They are medicine by their very presence; each offers a uniqueness that one comes to know through experiencing it. Each herb has its own particular cycles that merge with cycles of birds, bees, bugs and butterflies.

These plants can help heal what ails our Earth as well as what ails the gardener. We are losing diversity at an alarming speed, thanks to an agriculture that relies on poisons to grow food. These plants are champions at attracting pollinators, not only during flowering but also at seed production.

And the beauty of the plants themselves is something to behold again and again, through leaf, flower and seed.

These herbs lend themselves admirably to being grown in community as well as individual gardens, because they require little space. People working together could create productive herbal medicine gardens on school or church grounds, in public parks, in allotment gardens or on private property.

Because the healing constituents of herbs are so concentrated, relatively few plants can provide medicine for many people each year. Once the plants in this book establish themselves, they require little care or attention. Most can be divided annually to quickly become established plants elsewhere.

We hope that this book serves as an enticing and enriching introduction to growing, using, enjoying and benefiting from these wonderful herbs. Seeds and tinctures of most of them are available through the website of our company, Salt Spring Seeds (saltspringseeds.com).

Arnica

Arnica montana (Asteraceae)

Many Salt Spring Seeds customers have been surprised to learn that they can easily grow Arnica in their gardens. Arnica is usually thought of as an alpine plant, but we have been growing it successfully near sea level for many years.

Arnica is a low-growing, daisy-like perennial with vibrant yellow flowers on long stems. It makes cheery summer displays. It is sometimes called Leopard's Bane, Wolf's Bane or Mountain Arnica. Plants do best in full sun, with good drainage and acidic soil.

Arnica has been known for centuries as a very effective topical anti-inflammatory medicine and today can be found in all manner of salves, oils, ointments, gels and tinctures. People also use the freshly bruised plant or cloths soaked in Arnica tea. Arnica preparations can be applied as soon as possible to reduce swelling, bruises, stiffness and muscle aches from trauma or injury. Herbalists recommend it as well for hyperextensions, arthritis, bursitis and myalgia. It is also commonly found in homeopathic remedies. It shouldn't be used on rashes or broken skin and is toxic if taken internally.

It's very easy to gather Arnica seeds after the flowers are spent, but you have to be sure to get them before the wind blows them away. To facilitate separating the fluff from the seed, let them dry thoroughly for at least a few days on the bottom of a bucket in a warm place with a screen over the top.

Arnica seeds can be direct-sown in early spring or late fall but are best started in flats of potting soil in early spring. Seeds should be barely covered and will germinate in one to three weeks. The seedlings are quite small and slow growing at first. After six to

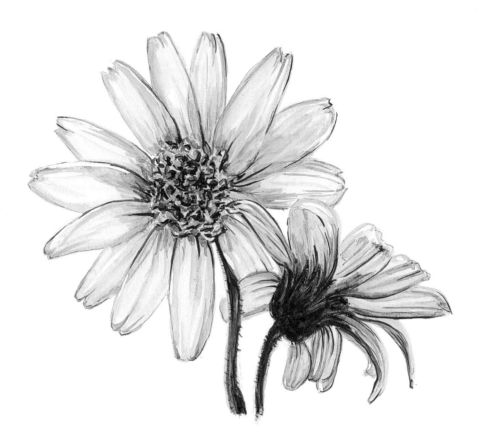

eight weeks, they can be put in their own pots to be later transplanted out to about a foot apart.

Once plants are established, it is quite easy to divide the underground creepers to multiply your plants or to help someone quickly establish their own Arnica patch.

Ashwagandha

Withania somnifera (Solanaceae)

A perennial shrub belonging to the Nightshade (Solanaceae) family and native to the dry regions of India, northern Africa and the Middle East, Ashwagandha can be grown in milder temperate climates as an annual or overwintered with care.

Start seeds indoors or in the greenhouse in early spring with bottom heat. Germination takes a week or two. When an inch high, prick out the seedlings and pot them up. At the end of spring, plant them a foot or more apart in the hottest spot of the garden. Ashwagandha loves heat and full sun. It tolerates most soils but prefers fast-draining, alkaline ones. The plants appreciate the addition of ground limestone to the soil.

Ashwagandha grows 2 to 4 feet tall, with oval leaves and yellow flowers, the latter eventually producing lantern-like pods enclosing pea-sized berries, which ripen from green to bright red/orange. Once ripe, the berries can be harvested for the tiny seeds inside.

Because freezing lessens the medicinal power of the roots, they are harvested with the first mild frost. Mulching with straw or leaves can be beneficial.

The adaptogenic properties of Ashwagandha have been used in Indian Ayurvedic medicine for nearly five thousand years. (Herbs that are "adaptogens" normalize and regulate the systems of the body.) A powerful antioxidant, it is known to strengthen the immune system after illness, chemotherapy or surgery. It is often referred to as "Indian Ginseng" because of its similar restorative and rejuvenating properties, although the two plants are botanically unrelated.

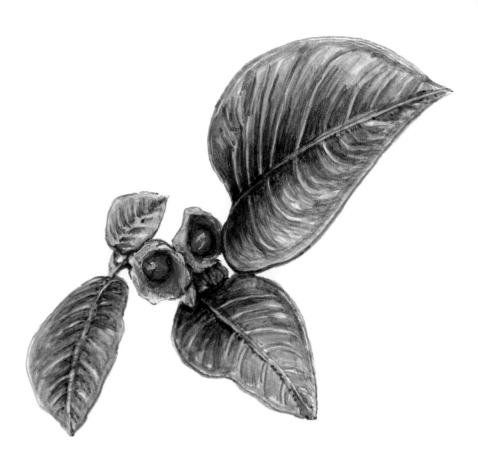

In Sanskrit, *ashwa* means "horse" and *gandha* "sweat" or "smell of perspiration," referring not only to the smell of the freshly harvested root, but also to the idea that the herb has the potential to impart the strength and vigour of a horse.

The Kama Sutra, the primary Sanskrit work on human sexuality, describes Ashwagandha as an herb that can heighten sexual experience, restore sexual health and improve overall vitality.

It is highly effective in reducing stress and anxiety, helping with insomnia and regulating sleep.

Astragalus

Astragalus membranaceus (Leguminosae)

Astragalus has been a highly revered herb in Chinese medicine for thousands of years. It is known as Huang Qi.

Preparations of its root provide a lifting energy that helps build resistance to weakness and disease. Its warming properties help tone the spleen, kidneys, lungs and blood. It balances the energy of all internal organs, improves digestion and protects the liver from toxic compounds. Laboratory and clinical studies confirm its abilities to stimulate the immune system, fighting bacteria, viruses and inflammation and helping patients who are undergoing chemotherapy and radiation treatments.

This premier Chinese medicinal herb has been said to build a protective shield around the body just below the surface of the skin that keeps out cold and dampness. There are no warnings about side effects in the literature.

Astragalus is rapidly gaining popularity in North America and is often included in blends with other medicinals to promote recovery in times of stress or illness.

In China, Astragalus is found along forest margins, shrub thickets and open woods. It is a perennial that grows to 4 feet, with delicate yellow, pea-like flowers from midsummer through fall. It does not like "wet feet" but prefers dry sandy soil in full sun or partial shade.

Many sources for growing Astragalus recommend two to three weeks' cold conditioning in the refrigerator and then scarifying the tough seed coat with fine sandpaper to facilitate water absorption and germination. We have often had rapid germination without doing either of these. Start seeds indoors in later winter, after

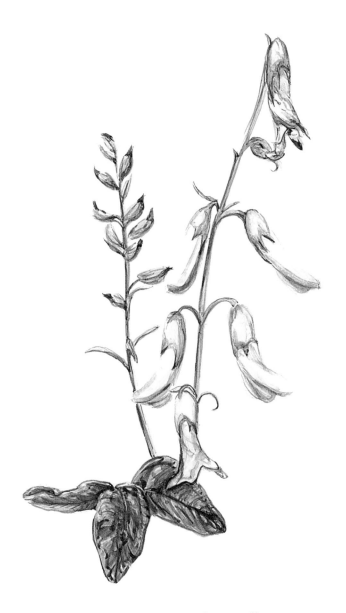

soaking them for a day or two. Transplant seedlings in spring to a little over a foot apart after danger of frost has passed. Protect well with a mulch of leaves, straw or hay for winter.

The roots are harvested for medicine when the plants are three or more years old.

Betony

Betonica officinalis syn. *Stachys officinalis* **(Lamiaceae)**

Wood Betony, Common Hedgenettle, Woundwort, Purple Betony, Bishopwort and Bishop's Wort are all names given to this medieval herb, which, in times gone by, was used in the treatment of a wide range of disorders.

Nicholas Culpeper, the esteemed seventeenth-century English botanist, wrote of Betony: "This is a precious herb, well worth keeping in your house."

It was believed that Betony was endowed with a power against the dark forces; hence it was often planted in churchyards and hung around the neck to drive away ghosts, demons and despair!

This hardy herbaceous perennial, native to Europe and northern Asia, forms a lush clump or mound of elongated heart-shaped leaves with toothed edges. In July, this mound gives rise to multiple slender, upright, purple-flowered racemes growing 2 to 3 feet tall, which bees just love.

Seeds can be sown in autumn or early spring, either direct-sown or planted in the greenhouse. Barely cover the seeds, tamp well and keep evenly moist until germination, which usually takes one to three weeks. Space plants 2 feet apart in a moist, well-draining soil in semi-shade to full sun. Once established, they can be successfully divided at almost any time of year.

Betony is once more gaining respect for its medicinal virtues. The aerial parts are harvested as flowering begins and can be used fresh (best for tincturing) or dried for later use. The leaves can also be employed to make a fine yellow dye.

A tea of the dried herb resembles black tea in taste and helps to relieve headaches. It has a sedative action, treating acute or chronic

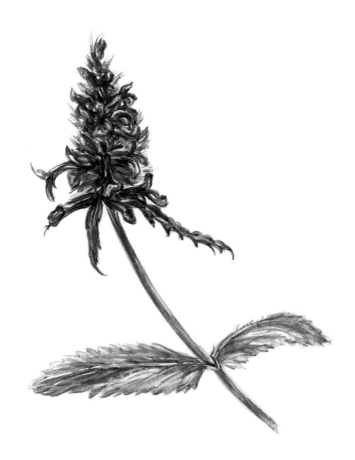

pain, frayed nerves, premenstrual complaints, anxiety and tension. It is also used in the treatment of addictions.

Betony is said to feed and strengthen the solar plexus, establishing groundedness, and in turn strengthens the digestive system, the central nervous system and various organs, especially the liver and gallbladder. Hence it has an overall tonic effect on the body and mind.

Externally, it is used as an ointment to treat cuts and sores. In homeopathy, a remedy made from the fresh plant is used in the treatment of asthma and excessive perspiration.

(Note: Do not take during pregnancy.)

Blue Vervain

Verbena hastata **(Verbenaceae)**

Not to be confused with its European sister *Verbena officinalis*, Blue Vervain is considered more striking in appearance and superior medicinally by many North American herbalists. Sometimes called American Vervain, Swamp Verbena and Simpler's Joy, it is a beautiful, hardy herbaceous perennial wildflower found throughout the continental United States and in much of southern Canada.

Reddish-tinted upright stems grow up to 6 feet tall, with long-stalked, lance-shaped, jagged-edged leaves. Long-lasting flower spikes bloom with multiple violet/blue flowers, attracting large numbers of pollinators from mid- to late summer. Flowering is followed by abundant, overlapping small brown seeds, which are best harvested with sequential shakings of the spike tops into containers or by cutting the seeding tops and hanging in a covered, dry, airy space over a tarp to catch the seeds. The seeds are a favourite bounty for birds and small mammals, so seed-saving can be quite the dance.

The flowering tops and leaves are harvested in mid- to late summer and can be used fresh or dried, in teas or tinctures. Infusions of the roots and seeds are also sometimes made.

Used extensively by Indigenous peoples as a nervine and antispasmodic and as an emetic for fever and stomach troubles, Blue Vervain is also employed in treating a wide array of ailments including flu, colds, headaches, throat and lung congestion, liver disorders, intestinal worms and irregular menses and cramps. It is an effective sedative and relaxant and is taken as a tonic for convalescence from acute diseases and in combination with other herbs to combat the symptoms related to menopause. Externally, it has been used for wounds, ulcers and acne.

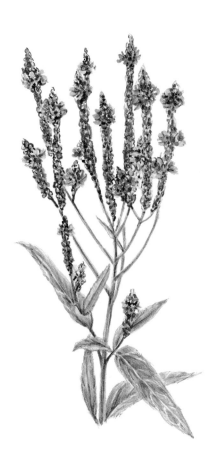

The seeds must be stratified before germination! Therefore, sow in the autumn or early spring, or cold-condition the seeds in a moist medium in a fridge (not a freezer) for two weeks. Then sow in a greenhouse or cold frame, barely covering the seed, and gently tamp. Germination can take between two and four weeks. When planting out, space plants a couple of feet apart in any moderately fertile, well-drained but moisture-retentive soil, with full or partial sun exposure.

(Note: *Verbena hastata* can interfere with blood pressure medication and hormone therapy, and large doses cause vomiting and diarrhea.)

Catnip

Nepeta cataria **(Lamiaceae)**

Catnip is justly famous for the conniptions it puts some cats through! Catnip tea is well known and valued for its relaxant and sedative properties.

Nepeta cataria is a short-lived perennial (usually three years) that is widely naturalized in North America. It grows to about 4 feet tall; blooms from late spring to autumn; and has oval, toothed, opposite leaves, a square stem and small, fragrant flowers that are white with pale-purple spotting.

Catnip grows well in the poorest dry garden soils, enjoys full sun but will tolerate partial shade and, like many other Mints, will become weedy if given the opportunity. Plants become more fragrant when grown in a sandy soil. Deer and rabbits don't like it, and it can repel certain insects, such as aphids and squash bugs.

Catnip is easily propagated from seeds or root divisions. Seeds can be surface-sown in flats or sown directly in spring or fall. Germination can be spotty and erratic.

About two-thirds of cats respond to nepetalactone, the active compound in Catnip, with behaviour that can include overt signs of affection, playfulness, relaxation and happiness. The effects are not achieved by chewing the plant, but by smelling the herb as a result of crushing, bruising or breaking its leaves.

Though mainly considered a feline euphoric, Catnip has a rich herbal tradition. Much like Chamomile, it has been used for headaches, stomach aches, colic and sleeplessness in children. It is an old home remedy for colds, nervous tension, fevers and nightmares.

Lemon Catnip, *Nepeta cataria* ssp. *citriodora*, is a plant that is very similar to regular Catnip but is a slightly smaller, hardier

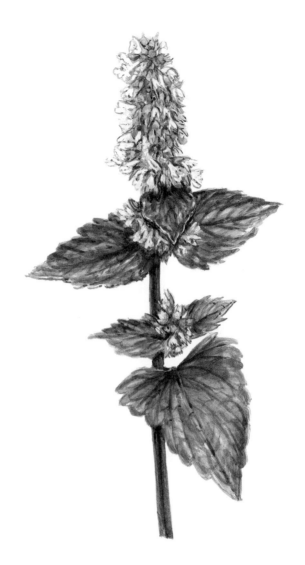

perennial that has a pleasant lemon scent. It is a good landscape plant. Some cats that will totally destroy normal Catnip leave Lemon Catnip alone. It attracts many pollinators and makes a much tastier tea, fresh or dried, that calms nerves, sinuses and colds.

To dry either Catnip for tea: Cut several long stems, bundle and dry in a paper bag. Crumble leaves gently and place in an airtight container.

Chinese Rhubarb /
Da Huang

Rheum palmatum **(Polygonaceae)**

Chinese Rhubarb is a truly striking herbaceous perennial, native to China and Tibet, hardy in zones 5 to 9, and grown in many parts of the world's cooler temperate climates. The sometimes red-tinged, large, angular green leaves and deep red / crimson flower plumes reaching up to 6 feet in height make this a focal point in any ornamental or herbal garden.

It is one of the first plants to re-emerge in the early spring, with its phallic flower plume pushing up, surrounded by rapidly growing palmate leaves. The plume height and the size and shape of the leaves distinguish *Rheum palmatum* from the classic garden rhubarb we eat, the latter generally growing to only a few feet in height.

Chinese Rhubarb is an early bloomer, flowering from May to June, with abundant small crimson flowers giving rise to multiple disc-shaped seeds. As the seeds dry and brown off along the length of the plume, watch for the first ones to drop; this is the indicator that they're mature and ready to harvest. Chinese Rhubarb is one of the first seeds of the season to be harvested in the medicine garden.

Propagation is easiest when done from seeds, as digging and dividing the root can prove to be quite a messy and tiring task! Spring-sow the seeds in the greenhouse. Bottom heat is not necessary, and germination takes around two weeks. Pot up seedlings and then plant out 3 feet apart into well-drained, fertile soil once the roots are robust enough to survive outdoors. It will tolerate

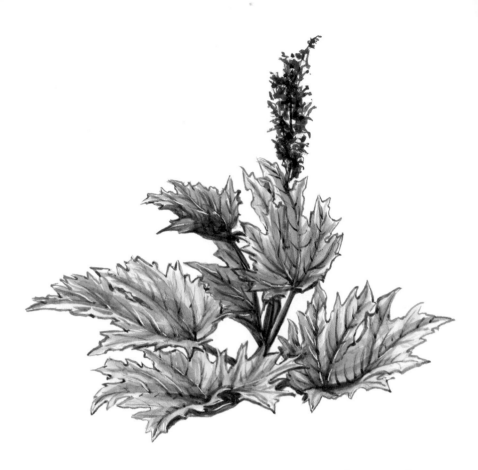

full sun in cooler climes but part shade in areas with summer heat, as too much heat can trigger early dormancy. The leaves generally start displaying palmate growth in the second year.

In Chinese medicine, Da Huang has been known for its medicinal properties for over two thousand years and is one of the most widely used herbs in traditional Chinese medicine. The dormant root is harvested at three years of age or older, thoroughly washed, then dried and cured. Revered as a safe digestive tonic balancing the whole digestive system, it is often used in conjunction with other herbs. Paradoxically, Da Huang has a constipating effect in small doses and acts as a laxative in larger amounts. Current research is investigating claims of its anti-tumour properties.

Codonopsis

Codonopsis pilosula (Campanulaceae)

Dang Shen, as Codonopsis is known in its native China, is a widely used herb in traditional Chinese medicine (TCM) because of its adaptogenic properties, which are similar to those of Ginseng, but milder. The lower cost and greater availability of codonopsis root has led to it becoming the standard replacement for Ginseng in many TCM formulas, earning it the name "Poor Man's Ginseng."

This vining, herbaceous perennial can grow to upward of 7 feet in height, prefers full sun to part shade and definitely requires something to twine around and climb. In flower from June to August, it produces beautiful five-pointed, violet-streaked, bell-shaped green flowers, giving rise to seed heads from August to September that are full of tiny red/brown seeds. The plant prefers slightly acidic, moderately fertile and fairly well-drained soils but is not drought-tolerant. It is frost-hardy down to -22°F (-30°C)!

Codonopsis seeds are best sown in the early spring or late autumn/early winter, as they benefit from a cold spell to break their dormancy. When the seedlings are large enough to handle, prick them out and pot them up, overwintering them in the greenhouse for their first winter and planting them out in mid-spring.

The roots are carrot-shaped or cylindrical, sometimes branched, and up to a foot long by an inch or more wide. When at least three seasons old, the roots are harvested in the autumn after the aerial parts have died down and the plant is dormant. The roots can be used fresh or dried and are rich in trace elements and 17 different amino acids, plus saccharides, glycosides and alkaloids.

The herb root is crunchy, sweet, warm and soothing. Taken as a gentle tonic, it increases energy levels, helps the body adapt to

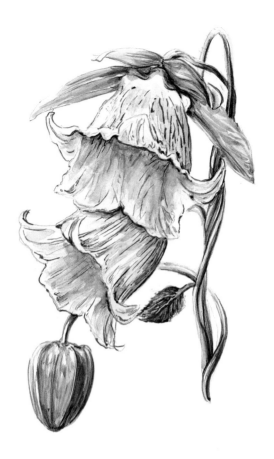

stress, tones the blood, builds Chi and strengthens the immune system. It invigorates the spleen and lungs, lowers blood pressure and is used to treat a variety of disorders, including memory loss and insomnia, anemia, shallow and strained breathing, poor appetite and digestion, and debility after illness.

Research has shown that Codonopsis increases hemoglobin and red-blood-cell levels, helping to reduce the side effects of chemotherapy and other medical treatments that utilize powerful chemicals and drugs.

Dandelion

Taraxacum officinale (Asteraceae)

Often maligned as persistent garden weeds, Dandelions could and should have a place in gardens instead. They are a stellar food and medicine.

Dandelions are one of nature's best blood tonics. Their greens have been found to have a pronounced stimulating effect on the digestive system, liver, kidneys and bowels. They contain large amounts of vitamins B, C and E, plus 10 times the vitamin A found in carrots. Adding chopped greens to your salads can save you a lot of money spent on vitamin pills!

The leaves can also be steamed or added to soups. The dried leaves can be used to make tea or herb beer. The flowers can be used to decorate or flavour various cooked dishes or to make wine.

The roots of Dandelion can be chopped small, roasted and boiled to make a delicious, full-bodied beverage. Allowing the roots to become slightly burned in the process sweetens the result most pleasantly. Substituting the grounding mellowness of Dandelion coffee for your regular coffee can save you a lot of jitters, as well as a lot of money!

Dandelions are one of the earliest, most reliable and most abundant spring greens, a crop you don't have to plan to sow and grow. But if you don't have them in your garden, it's easy to find seed heads and bring some of the seeds home to naturalize.

The seed heads are a masterpiece of architectural design. The seeds are easily plucked from their stalks in spring to early summer. They'll fly away if you're not careful. Put them in a container with a screen over them for a few days until they become dry enough to be rubbed from their parachutes. It's easy to establish your own

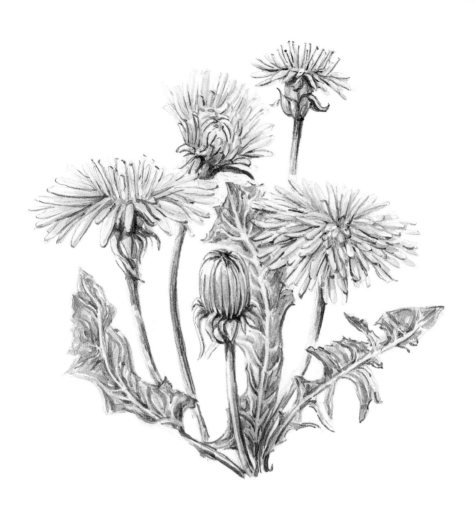

Dandelion patch by starting them in flats or sprinkling their seeds where you want them to establish themselves.

Aside from nutrition and medicine, the beauty of Dandelion flowers should also be more appreciated, perfect little puffs of sunshine that they are!

Echinacea

Echinacea **spp.** **(Asteraceae)**

Often called "Coneflower," Echinacea is probably the most recognized and important native North American medicinal plant. Growing in central and eastern North America, Echinacea varieties have been enthusiastically adopted into European, Ayurvedic and traditional Chinese medicine. The three most important species are *Echinacea purpurea, E. angustifolia* and *E. pallida*. It is commonly stated by herbalists that *E. angustifolia* is medically superior to the other two.

Echinacea's most common use is to treat upper respiratory tract infections. Trials have shown that Coneflower significantly reduces the length and severity of colds, and thus it is often recommended at the first sign of a cold. Recent research has found that it not only stimulates the immune system, but also reduces inflammation resulting from viruses. In fact, herbalists refer to Echinacea as the wonder herb for all acute inflammatory conditions, as it's generally mild enough to have no side effects.

Coneflower-root tea was used externally by First Nations to treat sores, wounds, burns and bites. It was considered a blood-purifying plant, and the root tea was brewed for acne, boils, canker sores and eczema. The root was chewed to relieve toothaches and to aid digestion.

Echinacea's flowers make a gorgeous garden addition. Coneflowers are stunning perennials and attract many bees and butterflies. Purple petals surround bristly orange cones on 3-to-4-foot stems. The orange seed heads turn black in the fall. Seeds can be harvested by cutting the heads, allowing them to dry for a week and then shaking them in a closed container to release the white seeds that look like little wood chips.

Echinacea is easiest to grow as transplants by starting the seeds in warm or cool flats in early spring. *E. purpurea* is relatively easy to transplant; the other two, especially *E. angustifolia*, don't respond well. Water well the first year, but, once established, Echinacea is very drought-resistant. Seeds can also be direct-sown in late summer.

Coneflowers can be grown in well-drained soil with full or partial sun. They tolerate poor, rocky soil but do not like wet, mucky ground. They bloom midsummer to fall and tolerate both heat and light frost. They should be spaced a foot or more apart. Cut them back in late winter or early spring when you're tidying up the garden.

Roots are normally harvested in fall of the third year. When making tincture, it is best to use the fresh roots quickly, ideally within 24 hours.

Elecampane

Inula helenium (Asteraceae)

Native to southern and central Europe, the Balkan Peninsula and central Asia, this giant, robust herbaceous perennial grows 6 to 10 feet tall. The soaring plant's main stem and branches are topped from June to August with long, slender, deep-yellow ray flowers, projecting out from bright-golden flower heads up to 4 inches in diameter. The large, elliptical leaves, green on top and fuzzy white on the underside, embrace the stem, becoming stalked toward the base, and can reach over a foot in length.

This hardy plant can withstand variable growing conditions, from partial shade to full sun, and grows well in moist, ordinary garden soil, though it flourishes best in a rich, loamy, damp but well-drained soil.

Sow seeds in the greenhouse in early spring, or sow them directly in the garden around mid-spring. They are light-dependent germinators, so sow them on the surface or cover very shallowly, so that light can penetrate. Expect germination within two weeks. After the second set of leaves appears, seedlings can be either potted up or transplanted directly into the garden, even if a few frosts are still expected. Plants may also be propagated from root stock offsets, harvested in the autumn, overwintered in pots and planted out the following spring.

To save seeds, pluck them from the top of the spent flower heads and let them dry until the small dark seeds can be easily separated from their fluffy attachments.

The octopus-like roots are large, fleshy and pleasingly aromatic. They are best harvested for their medicinal properties in the autumn of the second or third year of growth; after this, they tend to become woody.

Elecampane root has been used medicinally since Roman times. During the Middle Ages, apothecaries sold the candied root to soothe asthma and indigestion. Today, root preparations are used to stimulate digestion, kill intestinal parasites and soothe the stomach. It is an effective treatment for various pulmonary complaints, including bronchial congestion and infection, consumption, asthma and pneumonia. Elecampane also helps to boost the immune system, and research has indicated that it is effective against methicillin-resistant *Staphylococcus aureus* (MRSA).

For those looking for a great dye plant, Elecampane offers two distinct dyes: the root can be processed to yield a blue dye, and the flowers to yield a yellow / orange dye.

Fennel

Foeniculum vulgare (Apiaceae)

Fennel is a valuable plant, both as a nourishing vegetable and a medicine. It tastes great and is easy to grow. Originating from the Mediterranean, it can be grown as an annual vegetable or as a perennial for its foliage and seed crop harvest.

Direct sowing is best, as the seedlings don't take kindly to transplanting. Fennel prefers full sun with well-drained, loamy soil. Although relatively hardy, plants are liable to die out over the winter if the soil is not well drained or the weather is persistently cold and wet. Root divisions tend to take well at any time in the growing season, although they never seem as robust as seed-sown plants.

Growing up to 10 feet in height, with characteristic feathery foliage and yellow flower heads, Fennel is a striking addition to any garden and attracts a wide array of beneficial insects. It is generally a poor companion plant in the garden, inhibiting the growth of nearby plants, especially beans and tomatoes.

Late in the season, it's easy to harvest dry, brown seeds by rubbing them between your hands into a container. Both leaves and seeds make pleasant and soothing tea.

The plant is rich in B vitamins, calcium, iron, magnesium and manganese, and it has an extremely impressive array of medicinal qualities.

It has the ability to tone, strengthen, detoxify and heal the liver; it increases bile production, thus aiding digestion, and is widely used as a digestive and carminative. Fennel also has anti-inflammatory and antispasmodic properties, and so assists the immune and nervous systems. It is antimicrobial and has actions against a range of bacteria, as well as various fungi and yeasts. It is

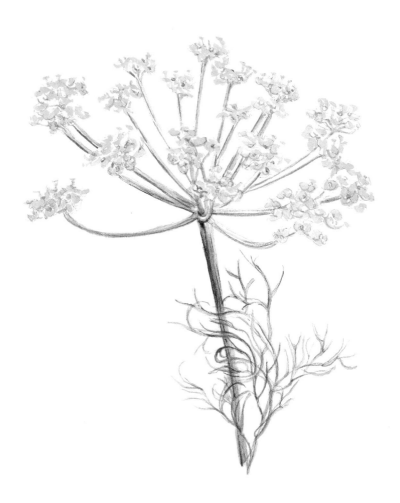

diuretic and detoxifies by stimulating the production of urine and the elimination of toxins through the urine. It is said to improve eyesight and is a galactagogue—i.e., it promotes lactation—and so can be extremely beneficial to postnatal mothers.

Syrup made from Fennel juice is used as a remedy for bronchial ailments and coughs. It helps to thin mucus so you can expectorate efficiently.

As a dye plant, Fennel offers up lovely pale yellows to forest greens, depending on the mordant and fibre you use. Overall, Fennel is an essential food and medicine to be grown in any garden.

Figwort

Scrophularia nodosa (Scrophulariaceae)

The small Snapdragon-like flowers of Figwort are quite inconspicuous: you'd never imagine that bees would love them so much. In our diverse gardens, the only other plant that comes close to attracting that many bees is *Phacelia tanacetifolia*.

Figwort is also a favourite plant of butterflies, hummingbirds and beneficial wasps. It is a widespread herbaceous perennial in the Northern Hemisphere that grows to about 3 feet in height in its first year and over 6 feet in succeeding years. It flowers from June to September, with the seeds ripening from July to September. Its leaves have a beautiful violet tinge when they first appear quite early in spring.

The name *Scrophularia* comes from *scrofula*, a form of tuberculosis of the lymphatic glands that Figwort was historically used to treat. The roots of Figwort have a long history of use for skin problems, sprains, swellings, burns and inflammation. Figwort is also a well-known remedy for sore throat, swollen tonsils and red, swollen eyes.

Also called Woodland Figwort and Knotted Figwort, it is a very esteemed yin tonic known as Bei Xuan Shen (*Scrophularia buergeriana*) in traditional Chinese medicine. Its roots are employed to "cool the blood" and to clear inflammatory and infectious conditions, including psoriasis and eczema.

Figwort is a very hardy, low-maintenance, drought-tolerant and rewarding perennial. As with so many plants, seed can be started 8 to 10 weeks before the last frost and transplanted out once the weather has warmed. However, as with most perennial herbs, it can be started at practically any time during the growing season and then placed in its permanent position before the weather turns cold. If started early, though, it will flower the first year. It is happy in full sun or part shade and is best thinned to 1 to 2 feet apart. It tolerates fairly wet soils and is hardy to at least 5°F (-15°C). Clumps can be separated and your plot expanded after three or four years. It is deer-resistant.

After the flowers fade, the Figwort seeds develop in teardrop-shaped seed capsules that brown and dry. They are easy to gather and clean. The seeds are easy to germinate as well but should be only lightly pressed into your starting mix.

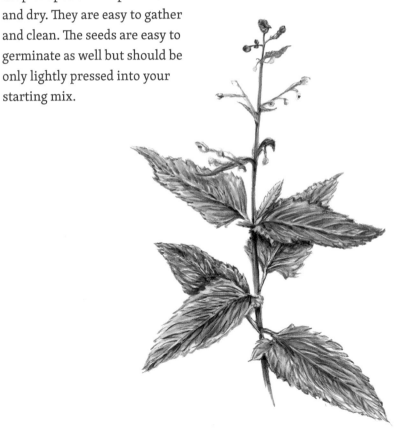

Greater Celandine

Chelidonium majus (Papaveraceae)

Chelidonium is derived from the Greek word *chelidon*, meaning "swallow," as Celandine generally comes into bloom when the swallows arrive and fades as they depart. It is also said that swallows use the sap to induce eye-opening in their chicks!

Swallowwort, as it is also known, has seen widespread use in folk medicine since the Middle Ages, with medicinal properties recognized to treat and clear eyesight, throat infections, ulcers and eczema, as well as colic and jaundice.

A native of Europe, northern Africa and temperate Asia, Celandine flourishes in the cooler parts of the year, preferring shade to part sun and moist but fast-draining soil, although it seems to be able to thrive almost anywhere. It can be an enthusiastic volunteer, so keep an eye out for its spreading habit!

This very showy, 2-to-3-foot, often short-lived herbaceous perennial, with slightly downy stems and abundant green/blue leaves, flowers from mid-May with prolific, attractive, four-petalled bright-yellow flowers. The latter are succeeded by long narrow pods containing blackish seeds, maturing and ready to harvest from mid- to late June.

The seeds are best sown in situ from February to May or August to November, covering the seed lightly and keeping evenly moist, with the best germination rates occurring when sown in the shade. Space plants about 18 inches apart.

The aerial parts are gathered when flowering and are best used fresh, especially when tincturing the plant.

In modern herbal medicine, the herb is used in very low doses as a mild sedative, antispasmodic and detoxifier. It relaxes the

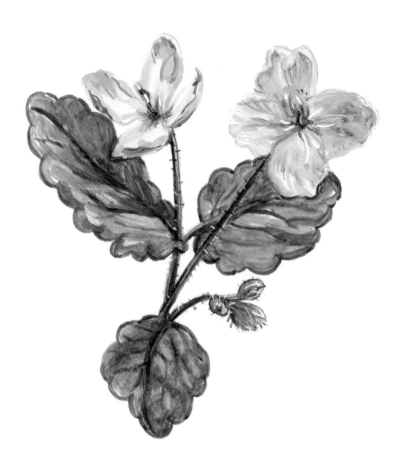

muscles of the bronchial tubes and hence is used in treating bronchitis, whooping cough and asthma. A weak decoction is useful for relieving stomach pains and inflammation of the biliary duct, helping bile flow, and for treating gallstones and jaundice.

When wounded, the plant yields a yellow / orange acrid latex, which, when mixed with vinegar, is used to remove warts, corns and skin tumours. New research indicates that Greater Celandine possibly has potent anticancer properties.

(Note: Greater Celandine is a low-dose botanical. Use with caution, especially when taking the plant internally, as it contains potentially toxic alkaloids. Do not use when pregnant or breastfeeding.)

Greek Mountain Tea

Sideritis syriaca **(Lamiaceae)**

Greek Mountain Tea grows wild at elevations over 3,200 feet in mountainous regions of Greece, Albania, Bulgaria, Iran and Syria. It is found in the rockiest cliffs of the mountainsides, where it survives with little water or soil.

Although it is an alpine plant, Greek Mountain Tea is an easy, carefree and pretty plant that makes a wonderful addition to an herb garden. It grows flat-topped and less than 2 feet high, producing grey/green elliptical leaves that are covered with a grey felt. Its flowers are pale yellow, lip-shaped and grouped together in long spikes; they last from June through August. They have a lemony fragrance and attract many beneficial insects.

Ancient Greeks used Mountain Tea as a healing and calming medicinal drink. Hippocrates, known as the father of medicine, praised its benefits for the immune and respiratory systems. For centuries, Greek shepherds in the mountains have brewed *Sideritis* for tea while tending their sheep, a practice resulting in the name "Greek Shepherd's Tea." Its taste resembles a blend of Mint, Chamomile and citrus. It can be brewed using the dried flowers, leaves and stems and is caffeine-free.

Greek Mountain Tea contains high levels of antioxidants, polyphenols and essential oils. There have been studies indicating its potential to boost immune response, aid digestion and act as an anti-inflammatory. Imbibers of this tea attest to its ability to reduce stress and anxiety. Recent research has even shown *Sideritis* extracts to be a promising preventive treatment for dementia and Alzheimer disease.

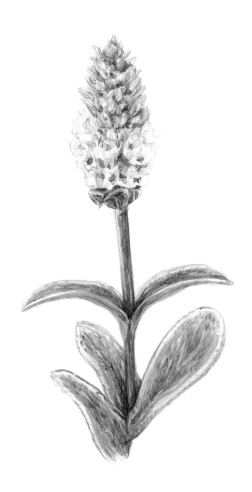

It is easy to grow this Mediterranean perennial from seed. Seeds can be cool-started in flats in spring, lightly covering the soil and transplanting out around mid-May. Propagation can also be done by taking cuttings. Choose a warm and sunny location, and it is okay if the soil is dry, nutrient-poor and very well-drained! Keep plants watered until they are established; after that, they require little care and are winter-hardy.

Greek Mountain Tea makes a lovely companion plant to other Mediterranean herbs, such as Thyme and Rosemary.

Greek Oregano

Origanum vulgare (Lamiaceae)

Greek Oregano has become well known in recent years for its antiviral, antioxidant, antifungal and antimicrobial properties. Oregano oil extract is widely available as a supplement and can often be found in pill or capsule form.

Packed with phenols known as thymol and carvacrol, this herb has been used to treat a variety of ailments since ancient Greek and Roman times, including indigestion, toothache and coughs. Folklore says it was created by the love goddess Aphrodite, who grew it in her garden atop Mount Olympus as a symbol of joy. It was commonly planted around homes to ward off evil spirits.

Greek Oregano is also one of the most familiar culinary herbs and an essential ingredient in Mediterranean cooking.

Oregano's fragrant flowers strongly attract pollinators and other beneficial insects, especially bees, butterflies and moths. It is a useful companion plant for most vegetables. It reaches about 2 feet in height and width, with soft, hairy leaves and flowers that bloom from midsummer to fall. It spreads naturally with underground runners and can even be used as a ground cover.

Greek Oregano is a very hardy, disease-resistant perennial. It is fairly tolerant of poor soils, strong winds and dry, hot conditions. Plant it in a well-drained, full-sun location for best results. Space plants at least a foot apart. Once they are established, allow the soil to dry out completely between waterings. This herb is easy to grow in containers, and there is no need to fertilize it once the plants are over 6 inches tall.

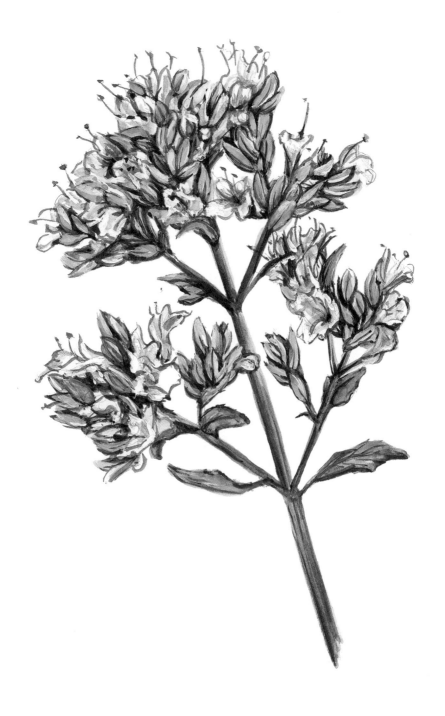

Gumweed

Grindelia spp. (Asteraceae)

Gumweed is a low plant of open places, found in dry, somewhat saline soil. In late July and August, it has bright-yellow flowers on rough sticky burrs. Each burr has five or six rows of very gummy bracts. Leaves are alternate, stiff and oblong. Lower leaves are gone by flowering time. Coastal species (*G. stricta, G. nana* and *G. integrifolia*) are robust and many-branched, while those found in saline meadows (*G. nana* and *G. squarrosa*) are spindly and less branched. Gumweed's daisy-like flowers are a special sight on rocky outcrops near beaches, where they appear to be growing in the complete absence of soil.

North American Indigenous peoples recognized the medicinal value of this herb. They made a tea from the resinous flower heads to relieve stomach aches, colic and indigestion. They chewed the leaves or made a tea from them for throat and lung problems such as coughs, bronchitis and asthma. The tea was also widely used as a wash to relieve itching and heal skin irritations. A leaf poultice or the gum from pounded flower heads was applied to Poison Ivy and Poison Oak rashes. This latter use of Gumweed has carried on to this day in commercially available fluid extracts of this plant. Herbalists classify Gumweed as antibacterial, anti-inflammatory, bronchial-antispasmodic and expectorant.

Gumweed is easy to establish in your garden. Seeds can be started in early spring and transplanted about a foot apart after about eight weeks. They can also be direct-sown when the soil has warmed up. Gumweed is a biennial or a short-lived perennial.

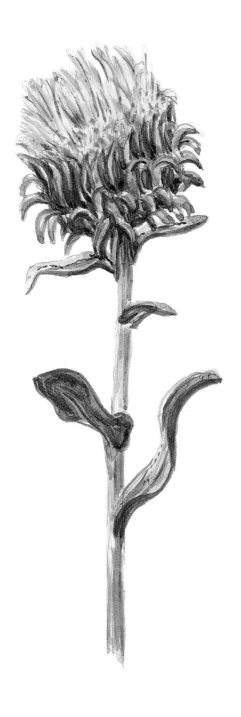

37

Gypsywort

Lycopus europaeus **(Lamiaceae)**

If you are looking for an interesting medicinal herb to plant in a moist area of your garden, Gypsywort could be the one. Common by the banks of rivers and streams, in ditches and in marshy areas, Gypsywort (also called European Bugleweed and Water Horehound) is an erect perennial plant growing 2 to 3 feet tall with deeply cut, pointed, hairy green leaves. It prefers semi-shade to full sun and blooms with whorls of small tubular white / pink flowers from early July to September, attracting large numbers of bees and other beneficial insects.

The leaves have an interesting aroma when rubbed, which some say is reminiscent of Hops. The plant is harvested as flowering begins and can be used fresh or dried, in an infusion or as a tincture.

It has cardiotonic properties, being taken to slow and strengthen heart contractions. It helps to ease irritating coughs and is useful in reducing premenstrual-syndrome symptoms and excessive menstruation. Gypsywort's main and increasingly important use today is in the treatment of hyperthyroidism. An extract of the plant affects iodine metabolism and the release of the hormone thyroxine, to the extent that it can help with treating an overactive or hyper thyroid.

Gypsywort is native to Europe and Asia and has the North American Bugleweed sisters *Lycopus americanus* and *Lycopus virginicus*, both of which have growing preferences and medicinal properties very similar to those of their European relative. Some Indigenous peoples used the North American Bugleweeds as an astringent, a mild narcotic and a mild sedative. They also used the

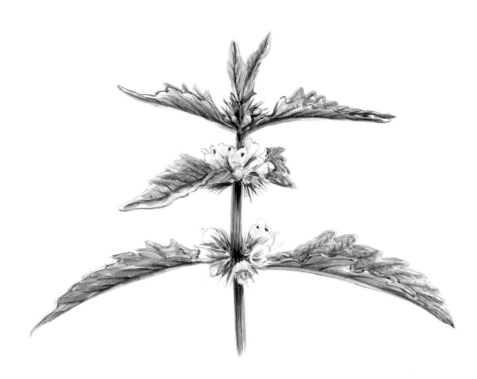

Lycopus roots as a food, digging them in the spring and eating them raw or boiled, or after cooking them in an underground pit.

The juice obtained from the plants yields a black dye that gives a permanent colour to wool, silk and other fabrics. The Romany people commonly used Gypsywort to dye fabrics, and it is said that this is the origin of its name. Today, the black dye is still produced from the plant on an industrial level.

Gypsywort is very late to go to seed each year but can be easily multiplied from its running roots, which spread in all directions, especially in wet soil.

(Note: Do not take if pregnant or if dealing with hypothyroidism.)

Hawthorn

Crataegus **spp. (Rosaceae)**

Hawthorn flowers and fruit are well known in herbal medicine as heart tonics. A tough, thorny perennial, Hawthorn grows rapidly once established and is happiest in an open, sunny position, where it can reach a height of 30 feet and a spread of 15 to 20 feet. Its dark green leaves are lobed and toothed. In late spring, it bears clusters of lovely, sweetly scented white or pink flowers, followed by bright red berries ("haws") from late summer well into autumn.

Seeds can be sown in late winter or early spring, or young shrubs can be planted from autumn until early spring. If you know of Hawthorns near you and want to start your own Hawthorn shrub or shrubs, you should pick the scarlet berries from the beginning of October onward. If you pick them too early, you risk the seeds being immature. Collect berries directly from the tree by gripping the branch and pulling the haws. In this way, no damage is caused to the parts of the tree that will continue to grow. It's easy to extract a few seeds from the haws and to start them in small pots with potting soil.

Hawthorn is said to slow the heart rate and reduce blood pressure by dilating the large arteries supplying blood to the heart. It has a gradual, mild action and must be taken for extended periods to produce noticeable results. Hawthorn tea has been used to treat kidney conditions and insomnia. Some Indigenous peoples consumed the haws in moderate amounts to relieve diarrhea.

Studies have supported the use of Hawthorn extracts for high blood pressure, angina pectoris and arteriosclerosis. People with heart conditions should use hawthorn only with a doctor's guidance.

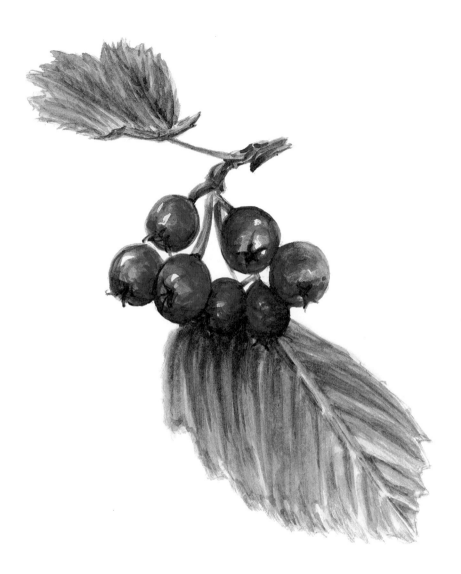

In Celtic traditions, the annual festival of Beltane, associated with fertility and passion, was held on the day of the first blooming of the Hawthorn. Now known as May Day, it is celebrated by dancing around the maypole.

Hops

Humulus lupulus (Cannabaceae)

Hops are the female flowers, also called the strobiles, of the Hop plant. Brewed as tea, they are the part of the plant that is so effective for insomnia, anxiety, restlessness and nervousness. It is hard to believe that Hops tea can bestow such a beautiful night's sleep while the Hop plant is such an incredibly energetic grower, often reaching over 25 feet in height in a season.

Hops are commonly known as a bittering, flavouring and stabilizing agent in beer. What is not so commonly known is that the relaxed feeling you get from drinking beer is not only from the alcohol content but also from the Hops.

The Hop has male and female flowers on separate plants. The male flowers are in loose bunches or panicles, while the female ones are in leafy, cone-like catkins, as in Lyn Alice's illustration. Thus, female plants are the ones usually sold at nurseries. The Hop plant is not usually propagated by seed but by dividing the young shoots from the main crown in spring, or by rooting cuttings from the older shoots and suckers in late summer.

Hops prefer a deeply dug, rich, moist soil with full sun. Although they are very vigorous, they can easily be trained over a chicken-wire fence or trellis to hang down at optimum harvesting height. Pick the strobiles in early fall when they are turning an amber colour. Dry them on screens or trays in a greenhouse until they become papery dry, and then store them in a cool, dark place for those times when you need to calm down.

Just three or four strobiles simmered in a cup of water for five minutes before straining will give the desired effect to most people.

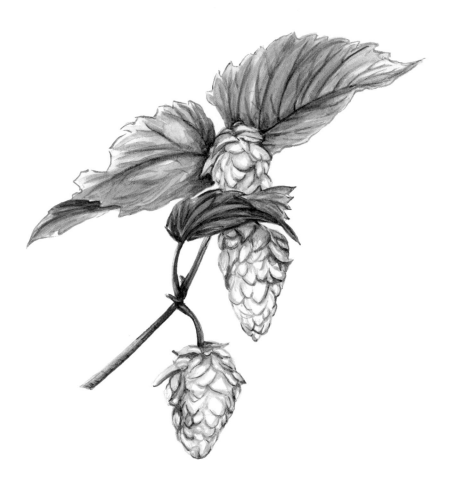

However, you should experiment with doses to see what works best for you.

No side effects, contraindications or adverse drug indications from the use of Hops are known. However, they do contain estrogen-like chemicals, which may be beneficial for conditions associated with hormonal changes, but which should probably be avoided during pregnancy.

Horehound

Marrubium vulgare (Lamiaceae)

A perennial of the Mint family, Horehound has leaves and flower tops that have long been used in home remedies as a bitter tonic for the common cold. Horehound has been used traditionally as an expectorant herb, helping to loosen bronchial secretions and to eliminate mucus. It continues to find a place in cough lozenges and cold preparations. It is also used for indigestion, bloating and loss of appetite.

Also called White Horehound, this hardy herb was employed in ancient Egypt, Greece and Rome and was very popular in Europe during the Middle Ages. It has also been part of traditional Chinese, Australian Aboriginal, and Ayurvedic medicine.

The Horehound plant is coarse and strongly aromatic and has square stems. Its broad, wrinkled leaves are woolly white below and pale green and downy above. The small whitish flowers are densely clustered and become burr-like seedpods containing tiny seeds.

Horehound is easy to grow, even in poor soils. It can be propagated from seed, cuttings, division and layering. Even moisture is important for sprouting the seed, which often germinates erratically. Horehound prefers full sun and a well-drained soil. Don't plant it in a spot that stays wet throughout the winter, and avoid planting it with herbs that need a lot of water. Space plants about a foot apart.

Once established, Horehound needs little supplemental irrigation. It is adapted to low-fertility conditions and, much like other Mints, can become invasive, spreading both by runners and self-seeding. It is easily grown in pots, and the home gardener needs only two or three plants for personal use.

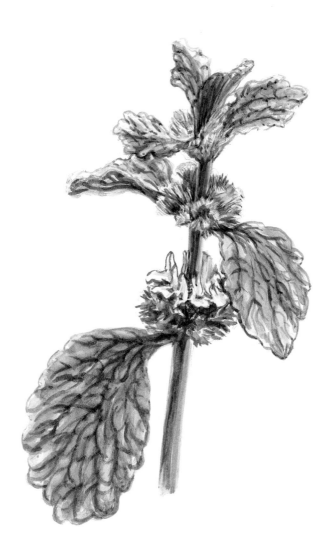

Horehound flowers are highly attractive to bees and other beneficial insects throughout the summer. At the same time, many pests, such as grasshoppers and aphids, are deterred by the smell of the leaves and flowers. Deer and rabbits don't eat it.

When using Horehound for tea, it is best to not use the bitter leaves fresh. The dried leaves take on a more delicious and smoother flavour. Simply pour boiling water over a teaspoon of the dried leaves, let it steep for five minutes and add honey for sweetening.

Hyssop

Hyssopus officinalis (Lamiaceae)

Like most of the herbs in this book, Hyssop is a hardy, low-maintenance perennial that attracts many pollinators and brings beauty to your garden.

Hyssop grows about 2 feet high, with slim, woody stems, narrow paired leaves and long, half-whorled spikes of little indigo flowers from June to October. It is quite an attractive plant. It is an excellent bee plant that deters cabbage moths.

Hyssop has a long history of use in medicines and teas. A strong tea made from the leaves and sweetened with honey is a traditional remedy for nose, throat and lung afflictions, and was sometimes applied to bruises. In the Middle Ages, Hyssop was a stewing herb. These days, it is used for flavouring meats, fish, vegetables, sweets and some liqueurs.

The leaves of Hyssop contain a volatile oil used by perfumers. Indeed, the scent of Hyssop leaves is possibly the herb's most stellar attribute. Just rubbing a few leaves with your fingers releases a spicy, minty aroma that has a very purifying effect. A traditional practice in Europe was to press Hyssop leaves and flowers into psalm books and then to sniff the pages during services as an aid to staying awake in church! Hyssop foliage was also strewn down the centre aisle in marriages of royalty to release its royal scent.

Hyssop can be grown in full sun or partial shade and does best in well-drained, somewhat dry soil. Unlike many other herbs in the Mint family, Hyssop is propagated by seed more effectively than by cuttings, layering or root divisions. Plant seeds just below the surface. They usually take two to three weeks to germinate. Transplant seedlings after 8 to 10 weeks, about a foot apart.

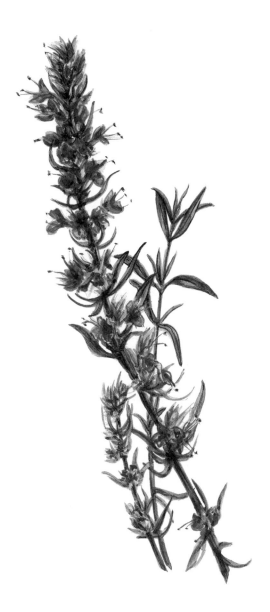

Hyssop requires little care once established. Trim back plants heavily in the spring and after flowering to prevent them from becoming too spindly and to encourage them to bush out.

Hyssop is not munched by deer or rabbits and is a pest-free ornamental herb that can provide pleasure for years to come.

Joe Pye Weed

Eutrochium spp. (Asteraceae)

Joe Pye Weed is a low-maintenance plant that is rewarding to grow for its impressive size, fragrant beautiful blooms and long history as a medicinal herb.

It is native to eastern and central North America and grows in roadside ditches, at the edges of lakes and streams and in wet meadows. Its leaves are in whorls of three to seven, and it can grow to 9 feet tall. The pink/purple flower heads consist of 10 to 20 tubular florets clustered into a broad, compact and very majestic inflorescence. The flowers have a light vanilla fragrance that becomes more intense when crushed. They last from midsummer through fall and attract a multitude of bees with their sweet nectar. Many gardeners say Joe Pye Weed is one of the very best butterfly plants.

Indigenous peoples used Joe Pye Weed for colds, kidney trouble and gastrointestinal complaints, and as a laxative and antiseptic. A poultice of its leaves was applied to burns. Joe Pye was a New England herbalist who used the plant medicinally, especially to help people with fevers. Another common name for this herb is Gravel Root, referring to its reputation for helping people pass kidney stones.

In 2000, Joe Pye Weed species were removed from the genus *Eupatorium* and placed in a new genus, *Eutrochium*.

If you desire to start this perennial from seed, store seeds in a sealed container placed in a refrigerator for at least 30 days, until you are ready to sow them. Direct sowings and fall sowings give the best results. When choosing a location, bear in mind that Joe Pye Weed self-sows vigorously. Press seeds into the soil rather than under it, as they require light to germinate. Joe Pye Weed prefers

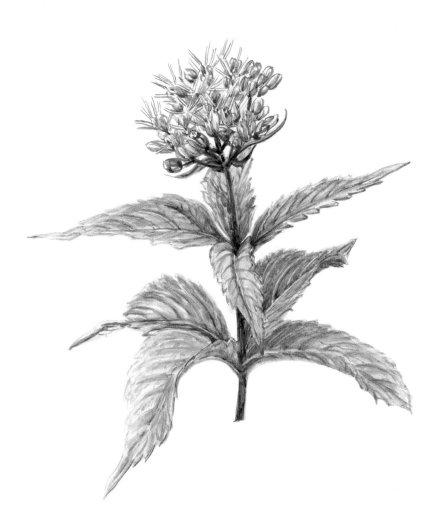

full sun and likes to be kept somewhat moist in average-to-rich soil. It makes a great background plant and needs plenty of room to grow. Plants need to be spaced a few feet apart. They can be divided in early spring after three to five years.

Joe Pye Weed serves as an excellent screening plant and a wonderful cutflower.

The flowers and seeds of Joe Pye Weed have been used to produce pink or red dye for textiles.

Korean Mint

Agastache rugosa (Lamiaceae)

Anise Hyssop

Agastache foeniculum (**Lamiaceae**)

The leaves and flowers of these two very similar plants make a fine herbal tea with a very pleasant licorice flavour.

Anise Hyssop's species name, *foeniculum*, derives from *Fennel*, another herb that has a strong anise-like scent and flavour. It grows to about 4 feet in height. It usually begins to branch when it reaches a foot.

Korean Mint is included on the list of 50 fundamental herbs in traditional Chinese medicine. It is called Huo Xiang and is said to relieve nausea, vomiting, coughs, fever and sore throat, and to work on the spleen, stomach and lungs. It grows to about 3 feet in height and blooms a few weeks later than Anise Hyssop—usually not until August. It is more strongly branched than its American counterpart.

Both Anise Hyssop and Korean Mint are short-lived perennials (two to three years) with abundant, eye-catching mauve / purple flower spikes and heart-shaped, toothed leaves. Like other Mint family members, they have squarish stems and opposite leaves, but unlike other Mints, their root stock is not invasive. Plants die back in the fall and go dormant in the spring. Both *Agastaches* are very drought-tolerant and pest-resistant. They are a special favourite of bees, hummingbirds and butterflies.

Gather mature seeds in the fall by tipping and shaking tops into a bucket. If they are surface-sown in potting soil and kept

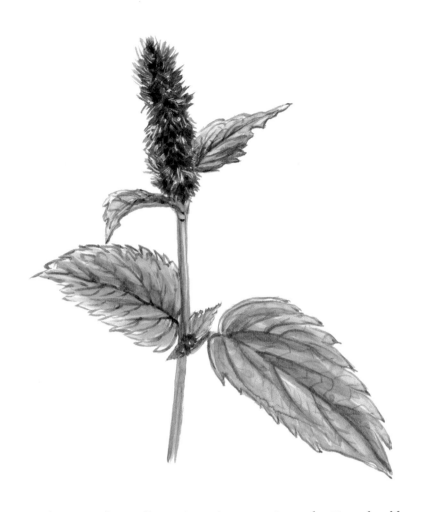

evenly moist, they will germinate in two to six weeks. They should be transplanted about a foot apart in a location where they can receive maximum sunshine. If started in spring, they should flower the first year.

Recent studies have indicated antioxidant, antimicrobial and antifungal possibilities for both of these *Agastaches*.

The leaves and flowers of Anise Hyssop and Korean Mint can be used to garnish fruit cups, iced beverages and other foods to impart an anise flavour. Individual flowers can be sprinkled on a salad or a stir-fry for a visual and tasty accent.

Ku-Shen

Sophora flavescens (Fabaceae)

Sophora flavescens, native to China and Japan, is an important herb in Chinese herbal medicine. Its dried root, known as Ku-Shen, has been used for over two thousand years to treat an impressively wide array of disorders.

Ku-Shen is harvested and dried in the autumn of at least its third season outdoors, at any time when the plant is dormant. Traditionally used for "damp heat" conditions, the dried root has antibacterial, antiviral and antifungal properties, as well as being anti-inflammatory. It has been used to treat hepatitis B and C and to help repair damaged livers. It is also effective against dysentery, jaundice, eczema, ulcers and trichomoniasis.

A decoction of the root or an extract made with vinegar can be applied as a topical wash to treat skin infections, inflammation and allergic reactions.

Growing 5 to 7 feet tall and 5 to 6 feet wide, this slow-growing deciduous perennial is, in cooler zones, considered an herbaceous perennial, as it will die back to the ground over the winter, whereas in warmer climes it grows as a woody subshrub. Long, arching racemes of beautiful cream-coloured flowers give way to clusters of very slender, bean-like seedpods 3 to 6 inches in length. The seeds are mature and ready to harvest once the pods start to brown in colour.

The plant prefers well-drained, moist soil and a sunny, warm position and needs protection from snow, ice and strong winds. As a nitrogen fixer, it improves poor soils, and it will stabilize loose, sloping ground.

The seed is best sown when it is fresh, or stored seed can be scarified and soaked for 12 hours in warm water, before being sown

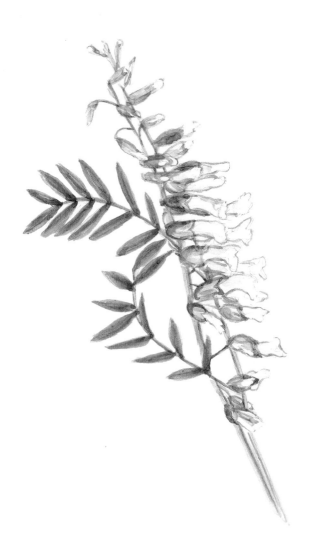

in late winter / early spring in a greenhouse. Prick out the seedlings into individual pots when they're large enough to handle. As they tend to be slow to establish, grow them under protected conditions until strong enough to plant outdoors in the late spring / early summer of their third season.

Overall, Ku-Shen root has amazing healing properties and is gaining wider recognition outside traditional Chinese medicine, with mounting research to support its traditional uses.

Lavender

Lavandula angustifolia (Lamiaceae)

A much-loved herb used since ancient Egyptian times, Lavender garnered its name from the Latin for "to wash." Among the over 40 different *Lavandula* species ranging from the Mediterranean to northern and eastern Africa and to southwest Asia and India, *Lavandula angustifolia* and its cultivars are the most commonly grown for their extremely fragrant flower spikes and the superior quality of their essential oils.

This perennial subshrub grows from 2 to 3 feet in height, with whorls of lavender blooms on flower spikes from June to August that rise above the narrow, oblong leaves. The flower spikes are harvested just as the first flower buds open, then bunched and hung upside down in a warm, dry, airy space for several weeks. The dried flower buds can then be used as is or in a tea or tinctured.

Lavender is antibacterial, anti-inflammatory and a carminative. It acts as a repellent to moths, flies and mosquitoes and has many culinary uses in salads, cookies, savoury dishes, ice cream and honey. The fragrant essential oil is how most of us experience Lavender, and unlike many essential oils, it can be safely applied directly on the skin. The oil is used to reduce the severity of headaches, migraines, muscular aches and pains and premenstrual syndrome, as well as to combat stress and insomnia. Also, its antiseptic properties help to heal wounds, burns, sunburn, scalds, bites and stings, and to prevent the formation of scar tissue.

Lavender attracts abundant beneficial insects; bees adore it, and thankfully deer don't! A sunny location is essential, as is a well-draining, sandy and slightly alkaline soil, the roots being susceptible

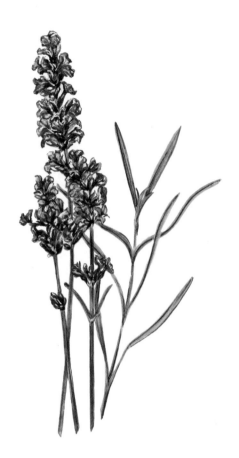

to wet rot. Drought-tolerant and somewhat cold-hardy (zones 4 to 9), the plants will benefit from a sheltered, south-facing spot.

Sandpaper scarification of the tiny hard seeds helps germination; then direct-sow in the fall or early spring in outdoor nursery beds or in flats of sandy soil in the greenhouse. Keep moist and cool until germination, which can be notoriously long, taking from two to six weeks. Pot up and work up into gallon pots, overwintering in the greenhouse, and transplant out the following spring, spacing 2 to 3 feet apart. Once plants are established, trim back a third of their foliage either in the spring or, preferably, in the autumn, which can help to prevent snow damage. Cuttings are best taken in late spring.

Lemon Balm

Melissa officinalis (Lamiaceae)

What would an herbal garden be without *Melissa*? Lemon Balm is probably one of the best-known medicinal herbs. The refreshing tea made from its freshly picked leaves is a common summer delight for calming the mind, lifting the spirits and comforting the heart.

Melissa displays the classic square stem of the Mint family members, with opposite, heart-shaped, toothed leaves. A very hardy, drought-tolerant perennial that grows well in sun to partial shade, it is not too picky about soil and requires minimal watering. The upright, branching plants reach 3 feet in height, with whorls of small white/cream flowers through July and August.

For optimal flavour and oil concentration, the leaves are best harvested just before flowering, in the morning after the dew has "burned off." Once picked, the leaves wilt rapidly and begin to lose their fragrance, so use fresh for salads, tea, tincturing and making essential oil. If drying the leaves, handle as little as possible once they're picked, making sure they are in a cool, dry and airy environment, out of direct sunlight.

Native to the Mediterranean and Eurasia, Lemon Balm has been in use since Greek and Roman times and takes its name from the Greek for "honeybee," *Melissa*, a being the plants attract in copious numbers!

Melissa's uses are many, from fresh leaf infusions applied to Nettle rash, insect bites and stings to soothe itching and reduce pain and inflammation; to tea or tincture for calming an upset stomach or indigestion, or to help with insomnia, mental stress, mild depression or restlessness. The essential oil is used as an insect

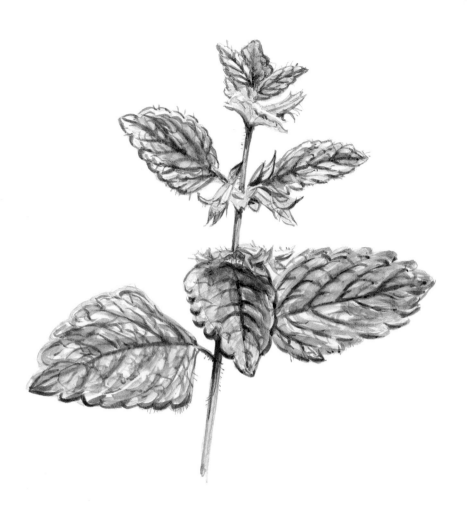

repellent or for its beneficial antiviral effects on cold sores, chicken pox and shingles. And it's effective in treating hyperthyroidism.

Sow seeds either outdoors in the fall or very early spring or in flats in the greenhouse after two weeks of cold conditioning. Some recommend light scarification of the seeds before sowing, although it's not essential. Barely cover the seeds, as they are light-dependent germinators; tamp down securely and keep evenly moist. Germination can be slow: anywhere from 10 to 35 days—be patient! Plant out 1 to 2 feet apart, being mindful that Lemon Balm will grow quickly and loves to spread.

Leopard (Blackberry) Lily

Belamcanda chinensis syn. *Iris domestica* (Iridaceae)

A beautiful addition to any garden, Leopard Lily (She-Gan) has a long history of use in traditional Chinese medicine. Native to Eastern Russia, China and Japan, it is not a true Lily, but a member of the Iris family (Iridaceae). The golden rhizome, harvested after at least three seasons in late autumn or early spring, contains several medically active constituents, including flavonoids, isoflavonoids and glucosides.

Acting mainly on the upper respiratory tract, lungs and liver, the dried rhizome of this bitter cooling herb lowers fevers and reduces inflammation and is effective against several bacterial, fungal and viral organisms. Currently, studies are under way to investigate its apparent potential to treat prostate cancer.

This hardy (zones 5 to 10) herbaceous perennial monocot prefers moist, loamy soil and full sun to part shade. From clumps of flat, sword-like leaves arranged in a fan growing up to 2 feet in height, upright stalks emerge from midsummer, bearing multiple short-lived (just a day) exotic flowers. These beautiful flowers are 2 to 3 inches wide, with six equally sized waxy yellow / orange petals with maroon / crimson speckles. The fertilized ovaries give rise to pear-shaped green seedpods, maturing to a fawn colour and splitting open to reveal the seed cluster that resembles a bunch of blackberries. It's helpful to stake the tall flower stalks, as they often flop or are blown over in strong winds.

Seeds can be sown in autumn in a cold frame, in the early spring directly in cool garden soils or by stratifying 7 to 30 days in cold, moist conditions and then sowing in pots or flats in the greenhouse. Be patient, as germination can take anywhere between two and eight weeks! Prick out and pot up the individual seedlings when they are large enough to handle. They can be planted out 1 to 2 feet apart in early autumn, to flower in the following season. If started in the autumn and planted out early enough the following spring, plants will flower that season. Propagation may also be by root division in spring or early autumn.

Be aware that slugs really love this plant and can destroy even quite large emerging clumps in the spring.

(Note: Should not be taken by pregnant women, especially during the first trimester of pregnancy, as this herb can induce the fetus to abort.)

Licorice

Glycyrrhiza glabra (Fabaceae)

Licorice, also known as Sweet Root, grows wild in parts of western Asia, northern Africa and southern Europe. It is a perennial legume that grows about 3 feet high and has an extensive branching root system, compound pinnate leaves that look almost feathery from a distance, clusters of small pale-purple/pale-whitish-blue flowers and oblong hairy seedpods that are between half an inch and an inch long.

Licorice contains a compound that is about 50 times sweeter than sugar. It has been used in food and as medicine for thousands of years. This medicinal herb acts as a demulcent (i.e., a soothing, coating agent) and as an expectorant (i.e., helps get rid of phlegm). Botanically, Licorice is not closely related to Anise or Fennel, which are sources of similar flavouring compounds.

In its long history of use, Licorice has been employed to treat a variety of conditions, including liver, circulatory and kidney diseases. As Gan Zao, it is considered one of the most important herbs of Chinese medicine and is frequently prescribed as part of Chinese herbal formulas. Around the world, it is used to mask the taste of medicines, as a flavouring agent in candies and tobacco and as an ingredient in cough lozenges and syrups. Recent research has shown that glycyrrhizin, an active ingredient in Licorice, can strongly impede blood clotting.

Licorice is an easy plant to grow, but it does prefer milder climates without extended hard freezes, and it can become very weedy because of its extensive root system and its ability to pop up 3 or more feet from the parent plant. It prefers good drainage, sandy soil and full sun. Start seed indoors around last frost and

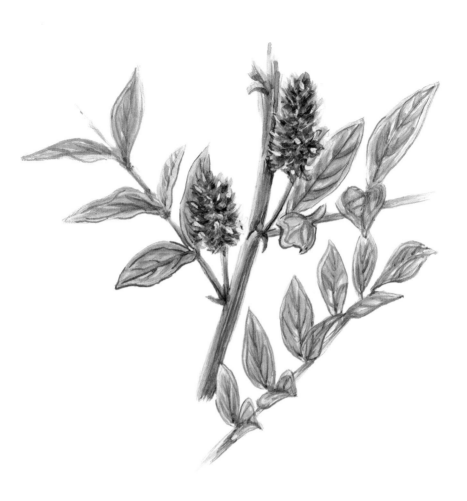

transplant out after about eight weeks. It can also be grown from root cuttings.

It is important to maintain soil moisture in the early days, but once established, this perennial is hardy and tough. It is usually pest- and disease-free.

Harvest Licorice roots in late summer after three or more years. Remove larger roots and replant smaller ones with growing points on them. The roots are fibrous and flexible and are bright yellow inside. Dry the roots for a few months before using them to make soothing and delicious Licorice tea.

Maral Root

Rhaponticum carthamoides syn. *Leuzea carthamoides* (Asteraceae)

Though relatively unknown in North America, Maral Root has long been used in Russia, China, Mongolia and eastern Europe for physical strength and endurance. Athletes use it to enhance sports performance.

The powerful benefits of Maral Root became apparent long ago, when Siberian hunters observed maral deer stags digging and eating the roots during mating season.

Recent scientific research is revealing that Maral Root stimulates mental as well as physical sharpness and fortitude. It provides relief from overstrained muscles, fatigue from overwork, and weakness from illness. It has become an effective medicine in the treatment of impotence and erectile dysfunction. As well, it helps people who suffer from anxiety, depression and alcohol addiction. It won't be long before Maral Root powders and tinctures are found in health food stores across Canada and the US.

In some of the coldest regions of central Asia, Maral Root has been used not only for fighting colds, coughs and sore throat, but also for endurance against extremely frigid weather.

Maral Root is high in antioxidants and contains ecdysteroids that help regulate protein synthesis in a way similar to steroids, but without their harmful effects. They promote lean muscle growth while reducing body fat. In herbal lore, Maral Root is termed an adaptogen because it increases the body's ability to withstand stress. It can increase blood pressure over time, so it's best to avoid long-term use.

Also called Russian Leuzea, it is a very long-lived perennial. (Some sources say it can live from 75 to 150 years!) Leaves are deeply

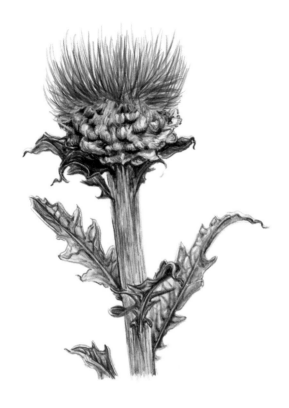

incised and pointed. In the spring of its second year, large, solitary, thistle-like magenta blossoms top 2-foot-tall thick round stems. One of the earliest spring flowers, they are loved by bees and have a wonderful vanilla-like fragrance. Maral Root would be a very ornamental addition to flower gardens, as well as to medicinal herb gardens.

Maral Root seeds are typically listed as requiring cold treatment, but we find that they are easily germinated indoors at cool temperatures: sow about an eighth of an inch deep in moist soil, keep soil moist at 50° to 65°F (10° to 18°C) and seeds will germinate within a week or two.

Marshmallow

Althea officinalis **(Malvaceae)**

Althea officinalis has been used from ancient Egyptian times through the Greek and Roman ages and into the present; the word *Althea* is derived from the Greek term *altho*, which means "to heal or cure." Historically, it was used as a poultice to treat wounds and bring down inflammation, and the nutritious root was eaten, along with the young leaves and crunchy seeds.

Most people associate the name Marshmallow with the soft, chewy confection toasted around campfires, not necessarily with the prized medicinal herb whose root was the original source of the sweet treat! The modern commercial candy no longer contains any part of the plant; however, Marshmallow is still regularly used by herbalists.

This hardy herbaceous perennial, native to most European countries from Denmark south, loves to grow in moist environments, from salt marshes, tidal riverbanks and seashores to moist meadows and the sides of ditches. Flowering to 7 feet tall with heart-shaped leaves and beautiful soft-pink/white flowers, often used in flower arrangements, the plant is covered with a velvety down that helps to prevent its pores from clogging in the moist nature of its preferred habitats.

Marshmallow has valuable mucilaginous properties due to the polysaccharide content of its roots and leaves. Plant mucilage is especially therapeutic for soothing irritations and inflammations, and Marshmallow is no exception. The roots, dug in the fall, are employed for digestive issues such as inflammation and ulcers. The leaves, best harvested just before the plant comes into flower, are used to bolster the urinary tract and lungs. A strong antioxidant

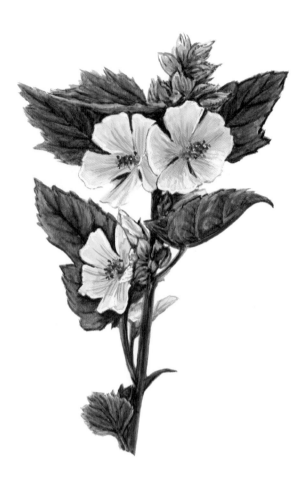

and immune stimulant, the plant can be used as a tea, tincture, poultice or powder.

Sow seeds in the greenhouse in the early spring; although some sources recommend scarifying the seed, it is not essential. Barely cover with soil, tamp down and keep evenly moist until germination, which takes between one and two weeks. Once the seedlings reach a couple of inches, they can be worked up in pots or transplanted out to a moist, sunny location. Alternatively, the seeds can be directly sown into a fertile garden bed and thinned to 2 feet apart. Spring is the time for propagation from cuttings and either spring or autumn through root division.

Motherwort

Leonurus cardiaca (Lamiaceae)

Wort is an old word for "herb," and this "Mother's Herb" is a beautiful perennial in the Mint family. It is a traditional female tonic from puberty to menopause and is also used for heart and lungs. Motherwort's botanical name means "lion-hearted"; many herbalists consider this plant one of the best for "gladdening and strengthening the heart."

Motherwort is a vigorous grower that can reach 8 feet or more in height. As with other Mint species, it has square stems and foliage that emits a pungent odour if crushed. It is sometimes considered invasive. Lower leaves have five cleft lobes with coarse teeth, upper leaves have three lobes and top leaves are oblong with one pair of coarse teeth. Plants produce clusters of pinky-white/purplish-white flowers that rise along prickly sepals and bloom from midsummer through early fall.

Motherwort is easy to grow from seeds, transplants or division. It adapts to most soils but prefers well-draining ones. If the plants are started from seed, it is necessary to cold-stratify them for a few weeks before planting. This tricks them into thinking they have gone through winter and the time has come to sprout. Broadcast seeds in late spring and very lightly cover them. They take about a week to sprout, and strong seedlings can be thinned to a few feet apart.

You can also sow seeds directly in the garden in the fall or start cold-stratified seeds in flats a few weeks before last frost. Motherwort grows quickly and spreads by rhizomes. Established plants can be dug up, divided and relocated in spring or fall during dormancy.

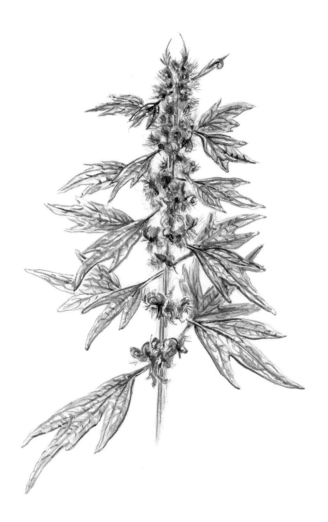

Once established, Motherwort is hardy and drought-tolerant and is rarely affected by pests or diseases. It is a great bee forage plant.

Motherwort has been used for centuries to regulate the menstrual cycle and to treat menopausal and menstrual complaints such as nervousness, insomnia, heart palpitations and rapid heart rate. It helps improve fertility and reduce anxiety associated with childbirth and postpartum depression, and it also promotes a mother's milk flow.

Mugwort

Artemisia vulgaris (Asteraceae)

Mugwort is native to northern Europe and Asia and can also be found in many parts of North America. It grows up to 12 feet tall in our gardens and self-sows readily. It has angular, reddish stems. The bitter-tasting leaves have a sage-like aroma and a dense, cottony underside.

When it is not in flower, Mugwort somewhat resembles Motherwort, and it shares some similar properties. Both are considered excellent nervines for treating insomnia, nervousness, hysteria and shaking. Mugwort, like Motherwort, has strong emmenagogic properties that can be used to lessen menstrual cramps and induce menstruation. It should be avoided during pregnancy and breastfeeding.

Herbalists use the tea or tincture to treat liver and stomach disorders, and Indigenous North Americans brew the tea for colds, flus, bronchitis and fevers; they also use the dried leaves for smudging.

It is sometimes called St. John's Plant, because legend has it that John the Baptist wore a girdle of Mugwort in the wilderness. It was believed to preserve the wayfarer from fatigue, sunstroke, wild beasts and evil spirits.

Mugwort has been used to kill parasitic worms, improve digestion and promote sweating. Leaves placed under pillows at night are said to induce vivid dreams.

In traditional Chinese medicine, *Artemisia vulgaris* is used in a therapeutic technique called moxibustion. A dried, cottony mass of it is burned directly on the skin to stimulate the immune system, promote circulation and relax underlying nerves. It is specifically indicated for conditions associated with coldness and deficiency.

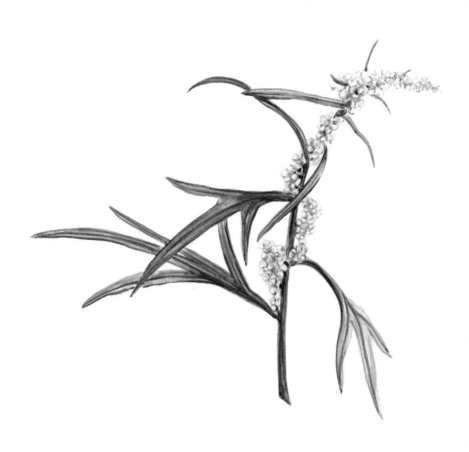

Ancient Romans planted Mugwort by roadsides so marching soldiers could put the leaves in their sandals to relieve aching feet.

Mugwort is commonly used in cooking to flavour foods and beverages, including fish, meat dishes, desserts, pancakes, soups, salads and beer. It was used in Europe to flavour beer long before Hops were employed.

Mugwort seeds are tiny, and it is best to start them in potting soil to be transplanted out after about eight weeks. Mugwort is known to repel moths and other insects. It is a hardy, attractive and carefree plant once established.

Nettle

Urtica dioica **(Urticaceae)**

Nettle is a very common wild plant that is often considered a nuisance when it should be regarded as a gift. It is a very nutritious food and a wonderful medicine. The first luscious-looking mauve/green Nettle leaves appearing on the edges of woods and moist damp places are a sure indication that spring has arrived! It is easy to start your own Nettle patch if you don't have access to one.

Many people know Nettle from the message of their small stinging barbs and are put off eating them for that same reason. But if you harvest the tops with gloves and steam them for a moment or two, they are delicious and there is no stinging effect at all. The first few weeks are the best, when the paired leaves of this perennial are often tinged a beautiful violet. They are a very rich green until the drooping flower clusters begin to form in late spring. Once in flower, Nettle leaves aren't nearly as special, though they are still edible and good for tea.

Nettle is high in chlorophyll, iron, calcium, magnesium and vitamins A and C. It is one of the few plants to contain vitamin D, which is necessary for calcium assimilation and bone development.

Nettle tea is soothing and healing when you have a burn, hives, hemorrhoids or kidney inflammation. Applying fresh Nettles (i.e., deliberately stinging yourself) will bring great relief from many kinds of skin rash and from rheumatism: the stings stimulate the body's blood flow and cortisone production. Nettle's high iron, chlorophyll and vitamin content makes it an excellent herb to take for anemia and other blood conditions. Nettle seeds are also packed with nutrients and contain acetylcholine and serotonin. They can be harvested in the fall after leaves drop off.

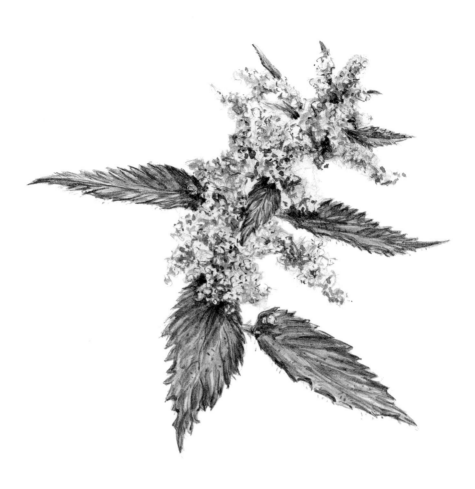

Massaging the scalp with a strong Nettle tea infusion or using it as a hair rinse after shampooing will improve the colour and texture of the hair and remove dandruff. Nettle stalks are widely used for making thread and cloth. The roots yield a yellow dye.

Orpine

Hylotelephium telephium syn. *Sedum telephium* (Crassulaceae)

Orpine is a succulent herbaceous perennial with many other common names, including Stonecrop, Live-Forever, Live-Long, Witch's Moneybags, Aaron's Rod, Purse Plant and Pudding-Bags! It is endemic from Asia to Europe and has been widely introduced elsewhere on the planet, particularly in North America.

Its fleshy leaves are a bluish green with hints of burgundy. Deep-red stems grow up to around 3 feet tall. These are topped with clusters of starry, showy, pale-pink to crimson flowers from July to August, giving rise to an abundance of tiny seeds from August to September.

Greek legend says that the son of Hercules, Telephus, used the herb to cure a battle-wounded leg that was not healing; hence its Latin name.

Orpine plants will succeed in most soils, sandy, loamy or clay, and will tolerate poor soils, although they prefer ones that are either dry or moist and well drained. It is drought-tolerant and hardy in zones 5 to 9, thriving in dappled light to no shade.

The plants are typically found growing on rocky or stony ledges in the wild; hence "Stonecrop," making them great for rock gardens and dry areas.

Propagation can be from root division or from seed sown in early spring through to early autumn. Orpine is an extremely forgiving plant to grow, earning the names "Live-Long" and "Life-Everlasting" because of the remarkable length of time it remains alive and fresh after being uprooted, subsisting on the nourishment stored in its fleshy leaves and swollen roots.

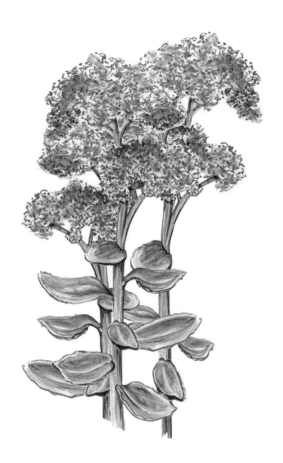

The leaves can be eaten raw or cooked or boiled in milk, and the resulting decoction taken to stimulate the kidneys. The plant is also useful in treating piles and diarrhea, and it has a growing reputation as an anticancer herb. A poultice of the crushed leaves has been used in the treatment of boils and carbuncles.

The roots can be cooked up in soups and stews, and the plant juice, mixed with vegetable oil, is used to heal burns.

On Midsummer's Eve on the British Isles, the plant was gathered to determine the future of love relationships; two leaves were placed side by side, and if they fell toward each other, the love was true!

Pasque Flower

Pulsatilla vulgaris syn. *Anemone pulsatilla* (Ranunculaceae)

Pasque Flower is an herbaceous perennial, native to Europe, that is otherwise known as Wind or Easter Flower or Purple Cowbell. It is a hardy plant, tolerating temperatures down to around -4°F (-20°C). The beautiful large purple flowers, which emerge early in the spring before most plants are stirring, will bring a smile to your face and make Pasque Flower an ideal companion for many early-spring-blooming bulbs. The flowers yield a green dye used in the colouring of Easter eggs.

Most of the leaves, covered with silky, silvery hairs, develop after the flowers, the latter giving rise to unique-looking feathery, silky upright seed heads.

Plants prefer full sun and dryish or moist but well-drained soils. Established plants are drought-tolerant. The seeds are sown on a moist medium, barely covered, tamped securely and kept cool and moist. Pasque Flower is generally a slow germinator, with results varying from 30 to 90 days. When the seedlings are large enough to handle, prick them out into individual pots for the first year's growth.

Good success comes from root propagation, taking root cuttings in the early winter and potting them up in a mixture of peat and sand. Initially slow growing, *Pulsatilla* can be a long-lived plant, the clump enlarging every year, with more showy blooms each year.

The plant is harvested soon after flowering and is slightly toxic, with the toxins being dissipated by heat or by drying down the plant.

It is a low-dose medicinal and needs to be treated with great respect! Taken internally, it helps in the treatment of female

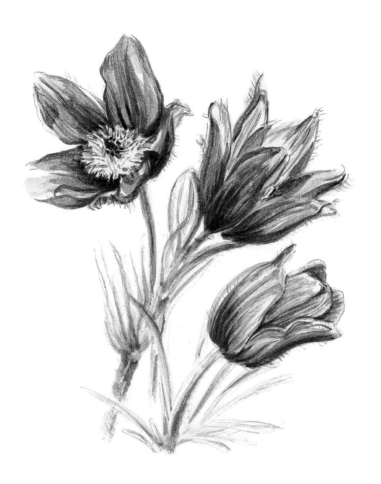

nervous exhaustion, premenstrual syndrome, inflammation of the reproductive organs, bacterial skin infections, neuralgia, tension headaches, insomnia, septicemia, asthmatic cough, whooping cough and bronchitis. The tincture is also beneficial in correcting disorders of the respiratory and digestive-passage mucous membranes.

Externally, it can be used to treat eye conditions such as cataracts, glaucoma and diseases of the retina.

The plant has become rare in its natural environment, partly because of overcollecting and habitat loss. All the more reason to include this beautiful plant in your garden plans.

Pleurisy Root

Asclepias tuberosa (**Apocynaceae**)

A beautiful, hardy herbaceous perennial, this species of Milkweed is native to the Prairies and eastern North America, common from Canada southward. It is often called Butterfly Weed or Butterfly Flower.

Growing up to 3 feet tall, with tresses of bright-orange / red flowers blooming from early summer to early autumn, Pleurisy Root makes a great ornamental plant in any garden. It attracts many butterflies, including monarchs, as well as abundant bees and other pollinators.

Plants prefer regularly watered sand or gravel soils (i.e., well drained) with full sun, although they can grow in light woodland and semi-shaded areas. They'll survive in low-fertility areas and will happily grow among grasses. Milkweed is hardy from zones 3 to 9.

The seed is a cold-soil germinator. If seeds are not being sown in the early spring, it is recommended to pre-treat them in the refrigerator (not the freezer) for two to three weeks before sowing warm. Germination is relatively fast and moderate.

Pleurisy is a deep-growing taprooted plant, so seeds are best sown in situ, in the garden bed, although seedlings and young plants will transplant, provided it's done with much love and care. Plants are best spaced at least 2 feet apart.

The tough taproot has a turpentine-like odour. Either fresh or dried, it can be made into a low-dose tea or tincture for treating a variety of lung conditions. Its specific action on the lungs makes it valuable in treating pleurisy, a painful inflammation of

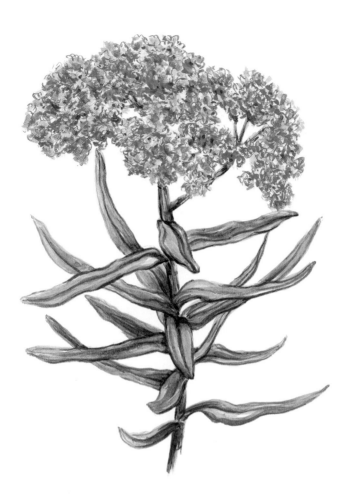

the membrane surrounding the lungs. It helps to alleviate the pain, eases difficulty in breathing and subdues inflammation. Overall, it has a mild tonic effect on the pulmonary system.

Indigenous peoples chew the root to treat a variety of lung ailments and boiled the root to aid in cases of diarrhea. A root poultice can be used for treating bruises, swellings and rheumatism.

The seed floss is extremely water-repellent and is used to stuff pillows or, mixed with other fibres, to make cloth. The floss has even been used to mop up oil spills at sea.

Red Sage

Salvia miltiorrhiza (Lamiaceae)

Also known as Chinese Sage, Danshen and Red-Rooted Sage, this perennial is an extremely important herb in traditional Chinese medicine (TCM), being listed in the earliest of Chinese herbal texts as an herb that "invigorates the blood." The red root is highly valued in TCM, and research both past and current confirms the validity of its use in the treatment of heart and circulatory issues.

A relatively hardy herbaceous perennial native to northeastern China and Japan, *Salvia miltiorrhiza* grows up to 2 feet tall, with dark-green, toothed oval leaves and flower spikes that rise above the foliage, yielding clusters of lavender/blue flowers throughout the summer. The long-standing racemes make it a beautiful choice for any herb garden in temperate northern climates. Bear in mind that the plant is hardy in zones 6 to 12, so if you're borderline Zone 6 and below, best to grow it in pots and overwinter it indoors.

Propagation from cuttings is generally successful at almost any time in the growing season, although plants grown from seed are hardier and more vital. Seeds are relatively easy to germinate, provided your source is no older than three seasons! Sow in the autumn or early spring. Germination takes from one to three weeks; bottom heat is not essential, though it will speed things up. Work up in pots and overwinter in the greenhouse before transplanting in late spring of the following year, spacing plants 2 feet apart.

Naturally, Red Sage prefers grassy clearings in forests, on hillsides and along stream banks. In the garden, it prefers full sun to part shade (and especially to full shade) and moderately fertile, fast-draining soils.

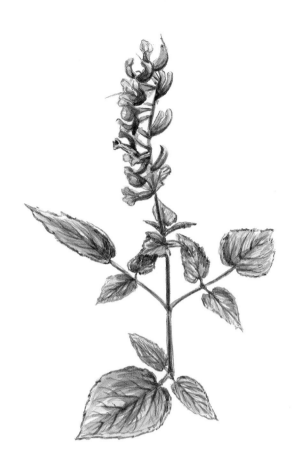

The red root is harvested at one year or older in late autumn to early spring, when the plants are dormant. Root preparations are traditionally used to treat circulatory congestion or stagnation of the blood, to help reduce blood pressure and to stabilize and improve heart function.

It is also effective in treating hepatitis and various skin diseases, including dermatitis, psoriasis and shingles, and is commonly taken for menstrual pain and as a sedative. It has antibacterial, anti-inflammatory and antioxidant properties.

The roots are also a source of the chemical compounds known as tanshinones, several of which are proving effective against cancer cells of various tumour types.

Roseroot

Rhodiola rosea (Crassulaceae)

Sedum rhodiola, Golden Root, Russian Rhodiola, Aaron's Rod, Arctic Root and King's Crown are all names given to this fleshy succulent perennial, steeped in folklore and revered by herbalists. Growing from 2 to 16 inches tall, with yellow flowers that sometimes contain red and purple hues, this plant survives in Arctic areas with ease and has to be one of the hardiest medicinal plants known.

It will grow in a variety of soil types, from rocky gravel and heavy clay to silty, sandy and peaty loam, preferring sun when grown at altitude and shade to part shade at lower elevations. It is hardy in zones 1 to 7.

Sow seeds in the fall or very early spring, as they need stratification of approximately two months at 40°F (4°C) or colder. Sow on the surface of a fast-draining potting soil, tamp down and expose to outdoor conditions—snow, rain and temperature fluctuations—all of which stimulate germination. If outdoor conditions are unavailable, the seeds may be stratified for 90 days in a moist medium in the refrigerator and then surface-sown in cool shade.

Prick out seedlings and work up in successively larger pots until the plants are a good size to transplant out, spacing a foot apart. They can also remain in pots to maturity with great results.

The young succulent leaves and shoots can be eaten raw or cooked like spinach and have been used like aloe to treat cuts and burns. The Inuit used a decoction of the flowers for stomach and intestinal discomfort and for treating tuberculosis. Viking warriors used Roseroot as fortifying medicine before going into battle.

There are a number of different ecotypes of *Rhodiola rosea*, all of which contain the immune-system-stimulating glycosides rosavin

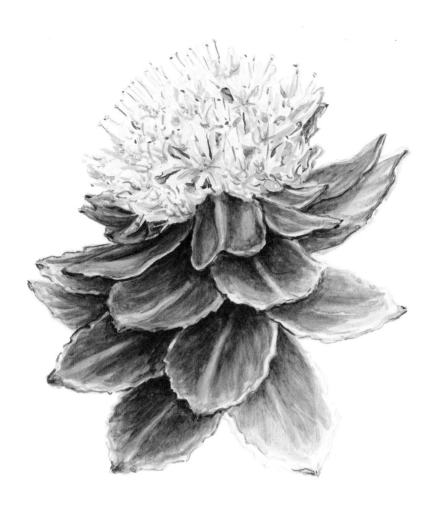

and rosin in their rose-scented roots, but in varying amounts. These glycosides can restore the body and mind after physical and mental exertion and stress, classing Roseroot as a true adaptogen.

The roots are harvested at a minimum age of three years, or, better still, at four or five years, when the root-mass increase gives rise to higher rosavin and rosin content.

Research has shown that the roots not only act as a general tonic but also improve learning and memory, combat depression, aid weight loss and inhibit cancer cells.

St. John's Wort

Hypericum perforatum (Hypericaceae)

This herbaceous perennial grows naturally throughout much of the world's temperate regions. Its growth habit can confuse some gardeners, as the plant displays two different-looking growth patterns. In the first year, it creeps along the ground, while in subsequent years, the plant sends up freely branching erect stems to a height of 3 feet, with abundant blooms from June until August. The first flowers commonly appear near June 24, the day celebrated as the birthdate of John the Baptist; hence the name St. John.

When crushed, the fresh star-shaped golden-yellow blossoms and flower buds exude a blood-red juice. When the flowers and buds are infused in olive oil, the resulting crimson oil, applied externally, helps to restore nerve tissue damaged by wounds, sores, ulcers, swellings and rheumatism.

The plant prefers a well-drained but moisture-retentive soil with full sun and is hardy in zones 3 to 7.

Seeds are best sown in spring on the surface of a sandy soil mix, keeping them evenly moist and in the light, as they are light-dependent germinators. Transplant or thin to 3 or 4 feet apart.

Pluck off one of the small, lanceolate leaves, hold it up to the sun and observe the perforated appearance of the leaf, implied by the name *perforatum*.

Be warned of the iridescent St. John's Wort beetle (*Chrysolina hyperici*) that can destroy plants in a season—two, if you're lucky! The beetle was introduced to control wild St. John's Wort, which is considered harmful to some livestock by causing photosensitivity, as it can in some people.

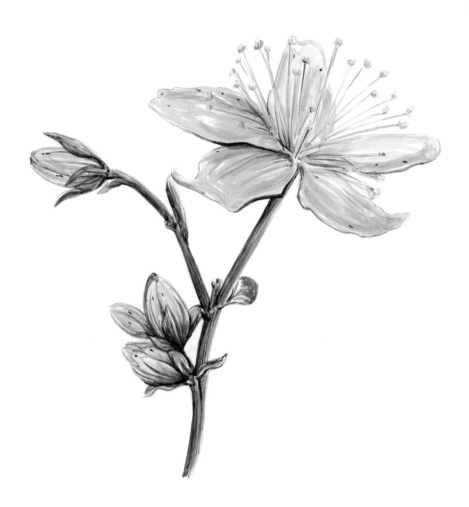

St. John's Wort has been considered a potent plant for over two thousand years, providing protection from demons and driving away evil spirits. Esteemed for strengthening the urinary organs, St. John's Wort has become well known for its antidepressant qualities and as an antispasmodic. Its antiviral properties are also recommended for treating some of the symptoms of shingles.

Be aware that St. John's Wort may reduce the effectiveness of a number of prescription medications, most notably the birth control pill, so consult your physician before using this valuable herb.

American Skullcap

Scutellaria lateriflora (Lamiaceae)

Baikal Skullcap

Scutellaria baicalensis (Lamiaceae)

These two well-known medicinal Skullcap varieties are not interchangeable and are used to treat different conditions.

American Skullcap, also called Blue or Virginian Skullcap, is a slender, heavily branched plant that grows 2 to 4 feet high. It derives its name from the cap-like appearance of the outer whorl of its small blue or purple flowers. It is a perennial native to North America that was used for centuries by Indigenous peoples to treat digestive and kidney complaints, menstrual disorders and nervous tension. Although Skullcap grew wild throughout Europe before the colonization of America, European settlers learned how to use it from Indigenous practitioners. Herbalists then brought it back to Europe in the nineteenth century. Today, it is used primarily as a sleeping aid and sedative, as well as to relieve tension, nervousness and irritability associated with stress.

Although the leaves and stems of American Skullcap can be used for medicinal purposes, they are best made into a fresh plant tincture.

Baikal or Chinese Skullcap resembles American Skullcap, but its blue or purple flowers are borne on single stems, and it is a shorter plant that is less than 2 feet high. It is the root of Baikal Skullcap that is used medicinally.

Baikal Skullcap is a prized Chinese herb known as Huang-Qin. It is used for hypertension, headaches, high blood pressure, respiratory infections, liver problems, dysentery and fevers. In recent years, it has become especially well known for its broad-spectrum antiviral properties. It is considered one of 50 fundamental herbs in Chinese medicine.

Both American and Chinese Skullcap prefer moist, fertile but well-drained soil in partial shade to full sun. Skullcap seeds germinate at a high rate naturally but do even better with a short period of stratification. Lightly tamp seeds into soil in flats and transplant after all danger of frost is over. Once established, Skullcaps are hardy in most North American locations.

Skullcap is easy to grow but does not transplant well. To increase plantings, divide roots carefully or take cuttings in early spring.

The deep-blue or purple flowers of both Skullcaps make them very attractive garden additions.

(Note: Both American and Baikal Skullcap should be avoided during pregnancy and breastfeeding.)

Valerian

Valeriana officinalis (Caprifoliaceae)

Valerian is the herb of choice for many people when they need to calm down for a restful night's sleep. Too concentrated a brew, however, could have the after-effect of creating rousing Technicolor dreams!

There are many different varieties of Valerian. One that grows in alpine meadows, with thick, shallow, winding roots, is quite different from the one usually grown in gardens, which has a concentrated root system. All Valerians, however, have roots with a very characteristic smell, an odour that some people love and others can't stomach. The flower scent is very different: quite fragrant and heady.

The stems of Valerian are hollow and grooved. The fern-like leaves are deeply divided and become progressively smaller on the flower stalks. The tiny flowers are white or pinkish, are arranged in flat clusters and start blooming in late May. Plants sometimes grow to over 6 feet in height.

The value of Valerian as an antispasmodic and sleep aid is well known, but it is not often touted as an easy and valuable plant for the home gardener. It's a very safe herbal tranquilizer and doesn't have narcotic after-effects. It can be grown in full sun or partial shade. It tolerates a wide range of soils, although it prefers a moist but well-drained loam.

Valerian can be direct-sown outdoors in early spring or started indoors four weeks prior to transplanting in late spring. Small seeds can be tamped into the soil or covered with a thin layer of soil. They should germinate within 7 to 14 days.

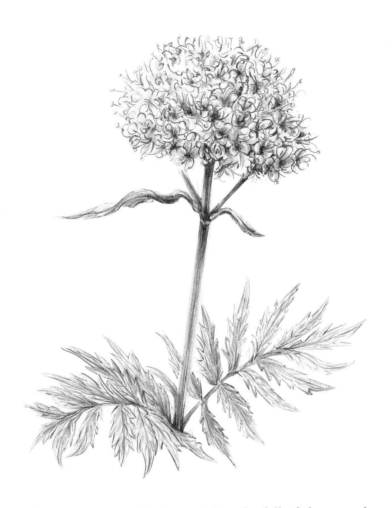

The roots are usually harvested in the fall of the second or third year. After removing dirt from the intertwining rootlets, cut them into small pieces and then dry them out of direct sun for about a week.

When you're brewing Valerian for tea, it's best to experiment to see what dose works best for you. A general recommendation is to gently simmer a small handful of dried root in two cups of water for about 10 minutes. That way, you can share the brew or reheat it for another night.

Vervain

Verbena officinalis **(Verbenaceae)**

Ancient cultures throughout Europe and the Middle East held Vervain in very high esteem. Its use for medicinal, ceremonial and superstitious purposes goes back thousands of years. The ancient Egyptians, Persians, Druids, Greeks and Romans regarded it as sacred.

Vervain makes an attractive garden plant, with deeply lobed and toothed leaves that are grey/green in spring, turning deeper green in summer. In late summer, pale-lilac flowers appear on tall delicate stalks. Plants grow about 3 feet high and attract many bees and butterflies. Vervain prefers a sunny, well-drained location and is very drought-tolerant once established. As with many of the other perennials in this book, seeds can be sown practically any time of the year, if you have a spot to maintain young starts before putting them in your garden.

Vervain is a prolific self-seeder; cut back plants before they go to seed if you don't want this to become an issue. After a few years, plants form clumps that can be divided and replanted. If you want to save seeds, they are easily stripped off the stalks late in the season.

Leaves and flowers are used fresh or dried for medicine. Plants will regrow if cut close to the ground.

Herbalists consider Vervain an excellent woman's herb, relieving congestion and cramps, stimulating menstruation, calming the nerves and lessening hot flashes. In general, it helps people wind down and calm down. In herbal texts, Vervain is classified as antispasmodic (relaxant), antipyretic (fever-reducing), astringent (constrictive), antibacterial and anti-inflammatory. Its astringent effect makes it a good oral rinse for bleeding gums, mouth ulcers

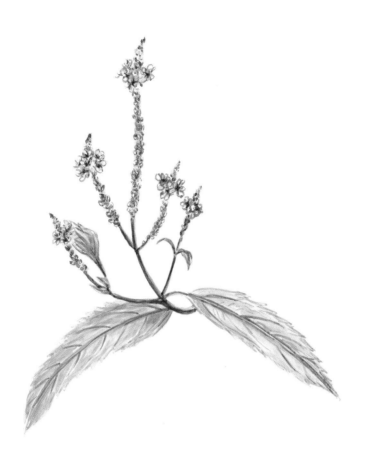

and throat inflammation. Its anti-inflammatory properties make it well suited to improve acute and chronic inflammation of the sinuses and respiratory tract.

Vervain is taken as tincture or tea, but the tea is quite bitter and takes some getting used to.

Vervain herb is sometimes confused with Lemon Verbena, which is an entirely different plant, although in the same plant family.

In Christian lore, Vervain was used to treat Christ's wounds on the cross, which is why it is sometimes called Herb of the Cross.

North American Indigenous peoples use Vervain as a natural treatment for headaches, circulatory issues and insomnia.

White Sage

Salvia apiana (Lamiaceae)

White Sage (also called Sacred Sage or Buffalo Sage) is one of the most popular, highly regarded and revered of all the herbs sacred to the Indigenous peoples of North America, with a characteristically sweet and powerful aroma. It is found in the coastal plains of California and Baja California and is traditionally used by the Chumash people as a ritual and medicinal plant.

This subshrub of the chaparral grows 2 to 3 feet tall with light-green/dusty-grey foliage when young, turning almost white as the plants mature. They grow rapidly during the summer months, putting out woody, flowering silver-blue spikes reaching 4 to 6 feet in height, with small white/pale-lavender flowers. This sacred Sage attracts many beneficial insects, especially bees; hence the name *apiana*, meaning "of or belonging to bees." White Sage loves sandy soil in a dry, sunny location and is drought-tolerant.

In autumn, after flowering is over and the seeds have been harvested, the leafy stems can be trimmed back, dried, tied into bundles and used for smudging. They burn with a thick, strongly aromatic smoke and are used ceremonially, often in sweat lodges, to cleanse the spirit and purify the surroundings.

Salvia apiana has antibacterial and antioxidant properties, so it is a great remedy for colds and flus, either as a tincture or as tea, or, because

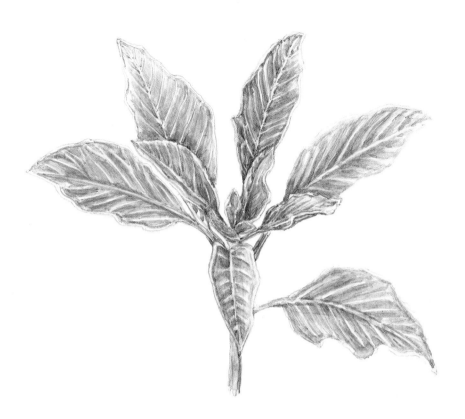

of its high camphor and eucalyptol content, as a steam inhalation bath to help clear congestion.

Seeds can be difficult to germinate, with rates as low as 25 to 30 per cent and taking between two and three weeks, often with flushes that can occur several weeks apart! Seeds may be scarified and then sprinkled over the surface of a predominantly sandy soil. Sparsely cover, tamp down well and mist daily in full sun or bright light at a temperature around 68 to 77°F (20 to 25°C). Be patient!

In zones 7 to 9, best practice is to grow *apiana* in pots and protect it from frosts; in zones 9 and above, they are best planted out on the south side of a building or solid fence, a couple of feet apart, and with a deep layer of sand surrounding the crown.

An extremely potent plant to grow and get to know!

Wild Bergamot

Monarda fistulosa and *Monarda didyma* (Lamiaceae)

Wild Bergamot is a beautiful perennial with bright-rose to purplish flowers, appearing June to August on unbranched stems that are 2 to 4 feet high. It is in the Mint family, and its mint fragrance is wonderful. Also called Bee Balm, it attracts many bees, butterflies and hummingbirds and definitely deserves a place in medicinal and wildflower gardens.

Monarda fistulosa grows in open, moist to moderately dry prairies, foothills and montane sites and is widespread and abundant as a native plant across North America. *Monarda didyma*, sometimes called Oswego Tea, is found in similar habitats, has a very crimson flower and is native mostly to eastern North America.

Bergamot, *Monarda didyma*, gets its name from the similarity it has in aroma to the bergamot orange that is used to flavour Earl Grey tea. *Monarda fistulosa* has an aroma that is more like Oregano.

Both *Monarda* species have a host of medicinal and edible properties. Bee Balm's soothing effect on the digestive tract helps to relieve indigestion, bloating and nausea. Its antispasmodic properties help to alleviate menstrual cramps as well as coughs. It has long been used to treat colds and flu. It has a gentle calming effect on the nervous system, which is helpful in ameliorating anxiety and stress, even in sensitive children.

In herbal books, you can find recipes for Bee Balm teas, tinctures, salves, steams, poultices, mouthwashes, jellies, vinegars and salad toppers!

Some North American Indigenous peoples perfumed their favourite horses with the chewed leaves of Wild Bergamot, and

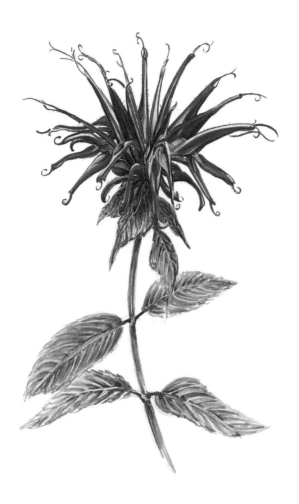

some used it as an insect repellent and burned it in smudges to drive insects away.

Bergamot is relatively easy to grow from seeds, cuttings or root divisions. It spreads via underground rhizomes and can become invasive in certain situations. It grows well in partial shade to full sun and prefers rich, well-draining soil in a spot with plenty of air circulation. Sow seeds in flats, barely covering them, from late February to mid-March, or direct-sow in early spring or October.

Bee Balm makes an excellent cutflower.

Wormwood

Artemisia absinthium **(Asteraceae)**

Famous for its use in the alcoholic beverages absinthe and vermouth (German for "Wormwood"), *Artemisia absinthium* has been known for its bitterness and medicinal qualities since ancient times. In Biblical days, Wormwood was a symbol for bitter life experiences, grief and sorrow as "bitter as wormwood" (Proverbs 5:4). Its bitterness was said to be due to the plant's absorption of human sufferings, driving sickness from the body and restoring peace and calm to the soul.

A hardy perennial native to the temperate regions of Europe and Asia, this majestic plant, with its soft lacy silver-grey/green foliage, grows from 3 to 6 feet tall, prefers full sun and dry soils and tolerates poor soils. It is great for rock gardens and provides a dramatic contrast when planted with dark-green-foliated plants.

A multitude of small wind-pollinated yellow flowers appear in July/August. This is the time to harvest the leaves and flowering tops that can be dried, then tinctured or powdered. Seed is harvested in the early autumn by shaking the dry browning branches into a large container and then screening and drying down some more before storage.

If starting indoors, seeds require light to germinate, so surface-sow by sprinkling the tiny seeds over a sandy soil mix in the early spring. If sowing directly in the garden, wait until the weather has warmed and the possibility of frosts has

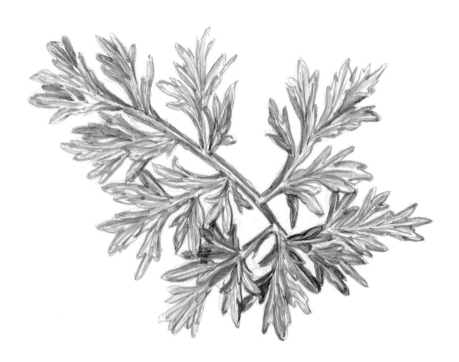

passed. If propagating from root division, autumn yields the best results, but spring will work too.

Many traditional bitters, aids taken before meals to stimulate digestion, contain Wormwood and prevent indigestion and flatulence. Wormwood is valued for its tonic effect on the liver and gallbladder. It is one of the oldest-known remedies for eliminating parasites and worms, especially roundworm and pinworm. It has anti-inflammatory properties and can be used for infections and to reduce fevers, and externally to treat sprains, bruises and lumbago. It is also a useful insecticide in the garden, and bunches hung in a chicken coup will deter flies, lice and fleas.

(Note: Extended use and high doses of Wormwood are to be avoided, as a buildup in the body of thujone, a terpene compound present in the plant, can become toxic. Also, avoid use during pregnancy or when breastfeeding.)

Yarrow

Achillea millefolium (Asteraceae)

Yarrow is very commonly found in open sites and in gardens and is one of the most widely used medicinal plants in the world.

It is an aromatic perennial herb with white (sometimes pink) flower heads and usually grows a few feet high. Yarrow plants are hardy, attractive and pleasant to have in the garden, though their creeping rhizomes can sometimes spread considerably. The abundant small flowers have a spicy scent and bloom from June to September. They are lovely in fresh or dried flower arrangements. The leaves are finely divided and look like large fuzzy pipe cleaners.

The genus name *Achillea* comes from the Greek hero Achilles, who reputedly saved the lives of many of his soldiers by applying Yarrow to their wounds. Yarrow plants contain alkaloids that have been shown to hasten blood clotting and suppress menstruation and menstrual cramps.

Around the world, Yarrow leaves have been commonly used in washes, salves and poultices for treating burns, boils, open sores, pimples, mosquito bites, earaches, sore eyes and aching muscles. Yarrow tea has been known as a tonic for colds and fevers because it stimulates sweating and lowers blood pressure. Herbalists classify Yarrow as sedative, antiseptic, anti-inflammatory and antispasmodic.

Yarrow leaves are sometimes chewed to ease aching teeth. Yarrow tea makes an excellent hair rinse.

When Yarrow goes to seed in late summer, it is easy to rub the seeds into a container. If you do, you'll find that Yarrow hosts an amazing number of small insects. Give these bugs a few days to flee and then put the seeds into a container. In spring, sow the seeds

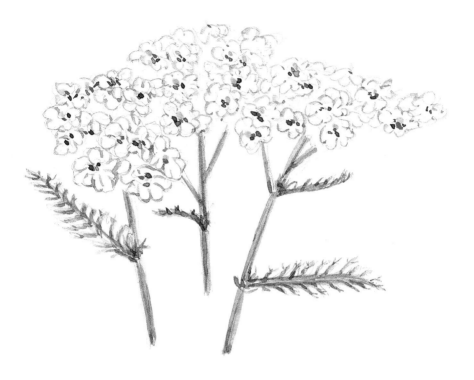

in potting soil and let them size up for about eight weeks if you want to establish a Yarrow patch. You can also propagate Yarrow by dividing the roots in spring or fall. It requires little care, is very drought-resistant and prefers full sun.

Yarrow is a significant healing plant that is unlikely to ever be on an endangered list.

Harvesting Herbs

Over time, as you continue growing medicinal perennials, you gain a deeper knowledge of the plants and develop stronger relationships with them. A large piece of this growth comes from harvesting and using the herbs. You begin to understand and learn the methods and amounts you can harvest in order to maintain the overall health and genetic diversity of plant populations. This practice of sustainable harvesting is even more crucial when you're working with wild populations, the consequences of your harvesting decisions having a broader impact not just on the harvested plant population, but on the overall health of the ecosystem in which they live.

When embarking on a harvesting journey, know beforehand what your intentions are in harvesting, whether from your own garden or from wild populations. Are you going to use the herb straight away, or is it going to be processed and stored? Either way, getting any equipment and/or the drying area ready before harvesting is a good practice and ensures you'll be using the herb in all its freshness. One thing to remember throughout the cycle of harvesting and processing is to label the harvested herb, noting whatever stage it is at!

Wildcrafting

When we venture out to Mother Nature to gather the wild medicinals she offers, responsible harvesting becomes a must. It ensures the health and longevity of the populations from which you are harvesting and shows a deep respect and reverence for nature. Many populations of medicinals in the wild have been dramatically impacted by overharvesting through wildcrafting, some to the point of collapse (Goldenseal, American Ginseng) and others to near extinction (*Echinacea tennesseensis*). We offer some guidelines to consider and hopefully practise as you step into nature and organize to go wildcrafting medicinals.

- Know the land where you wish to harvest—do you need permission from the owners, leaseholders and / or traditional keepers of the land?
- Correctly identify the plant (knowing the Latin name is important for this), and determine whether it's potentially poisonous and whether it's a rare or endangered species. Check in with unitedplantsavers.org.
- Know the life cycle of the plant you are harvesting.
- Sit with the plants, ask permission to harvest, leave an offering.
- Bring the proper tools for the job, as you don't want to unnecessarily damage the plants.
- Ensure that the plant population has not been exposed to chemicals, either through spraying or from other forms of pollution (exhaust, off-gassing from an industrial source).
- Always harvest from large populations—check the area for the largest and healthiest population.
- Harvest only what you need; take no more than 10 per cent.
- Don't harvest the elders of the population; they hold the best genetics for maintaining the population.
- Preferably harvest in good weather, as harvesting in wet conditions can damage the soil.
- Step lightly on the Earth, leave no trace, be undetectable.

When and How to Harvest

You want to harvest herbs at their peak of vitality, collecting material from healthy plants that are free of disease, insect damage and pollution. This is important; not adhering to it can lead to disease and decay in the dried, stored plant material. Wear gloves, especially when gathering from prickly or allergenic plants, and always cut with sharp knives, scissors or secateurs, causing as little damage as possible to the overall integrity of the plant. Harvest the herbs when the sun is not too hot, ideally on a sunny morning when the sun's warmth has evaporated the dew off the plants. Harvested herbs need to be as dry as possible, as surface moisture tends to encourage moulds—unless, of course, you are using them fresh!

Consult detailed herbal texts and resources to research each herb; every variety is unique, and different parts of the plant may need to be treated differently during processing. Getting to know the plants, observing and learning about them, is a joy.

Here is a rough guide to harvesting the various parts of medicinal herbs.

- **Flowers:** Harvest from summer through early autumn. It's important to know if the blossoms need to be picked in full bloom or at the budding/early-flowering stage. Remember, flowers give rise to fruits and seeds! Best not to harvest flowers before the dew is off them in the morning, on a rainy day or if it has rained recently.
- **Leaves and aerial parts:** Harvest from spring to early autumn, depending on the species. A plant's chemical constituents change as its priorities change throughout the season. It is often best to harvest leaves either prior to flowering or after seeding, when the new autumnal growth appears. Harvest

large leaves; smaller leaves are best left on the stem. Always look for healthy whole leaves, not ripped, discoloured, diseased or insect-infested.

- **Roots and rhizomes:** Harvest in the early spring or mid- to late autumn. Autumn is generally the best time, once the aerial parts have died off and the plant's vitality has been drawn down into the roots. Avoid harvesting in the rain or when the soil is too moist, as this can damage the soil integrity—and get really messy! Hose down the roots, and don't use an abrasive like a brush or scrubber; we don't want to damage the surface, as this can encourage pests and microbial spoilage.
- **Barks:** Harvest in the morning, either in the spring as the sap is rising or in the autumn as the sap is drawn down and there seems to be less bleed of the sap. Do not strip completely around the girth, as this will kill the plant. It is best to strip small vertical lengths.
- **Sap or resin:** Harvest either in the spring when the sap is rising or in the autumn when it is drawing down.
- **Fruits:** Harvest in the late summer and autumn as the fruits become ripe. A good indicator of ripeness is the ease with which the fruit can be harvested from the plant. Harvest with care, avoid bruising and process or refrigerate immediately.
- **Seeds:** Harvest throughout the summer and into autumn as the seeds become fully ripe, which can vary widely between different species. It's important to monitor the plants closely, as wildlife can seriously impact your seed harvest (i.e., eat the lot!), so be aware.

Once the plant material has been harvested, it is important to deal with it as quickly as possible, whether it's being used fresh or being dried and stored.

Drying

You've already prepped the equipment and drying area before beginning the harvest, so you're ready to go! Farmers, growers and herbalists use various techniques to dry down plant material depending on scale, but whatever techniques you're using, there are some basics to bear in mind when drying down your medicinal herbs for future use.

- **Airflow:** The more movement of air there is, the better, but not so much that it blows the plant material off trays or screens!
- **Temperature:** In general, the ambient air temperature should not exceed 100°F (38°C), as above this temperature important chemical constituents of the material can become damaged.
- **Light:** Generally, avoid drying herbs in direct sunlight; if possible, drying in the dark can really help with the overall quality.

If drying in a shaded outdoor area, remember that the plant material will likely pick up moisture overnight from natural dew, so it's best to bring the material into an area where this will not be an issue. Do not over-dry the herbs, as doing so can compromise their structural integrity and degrade key chemical constituents.

Some of the techniques used to dry down plant material are:

- Hanging in bundles.
- Placing on screens, racks or trays (with materials spread thinly and turned regularly).
- Using a dehydrator, at temperatures no higher than 100°F (38°C), as mentioned above.

Storage

The reality is that, once dried, medicinal herbs will naturally degrade over time. Generally, dried aerial parts have a storage life of a year, and roots, seeds and barks two to three years; seeds can be longer, depending on the species. Broken or crushed herbs lose their vitality more rapidly than whole, uncut herbs.

Here are some guidelines on various criteria that can help prolong the storage life and the integrity of your medicinals.

- **Containers:** Vacuum-sealed packaging is great, but not always available or practical. Use labelled dark-glass containers with airtight lids. Alternatives include new brown-paper bags and sealable plastic bags.
- **Labelling:** Include the name of the herb, harvest source and date of harvest.
- **Temperature:** Maintain a steady temperature. Somewhere between 41° and 53°ꜰ (5° and 12°ᴄ) is ideal.
- **Humidity:** The lower the relative humidity of the storage area, the better. Below 50 per cent is a good starter.
- **Darkness:** Once dried, herbs exposed to light can rapidly lose colour, vibrancy and overall quality.
- **Insects:** Hopefully, the drying process has done away with any potential insect infestations. Check material every few weeks to make sure!
- **Rodents:** Our rodent friends are always on the lookout for new sources of food, so rodent-proof storage is a must.
- **Freezing:** Generally, freeze-drying is better suited to culinary herbs than to medicinals.

These are some general guidelines to successfully harvesting, processing and storing your medicinal herbs. There are many great herbal books and websites that go into much more detail on techniques and methods, as well as on the specific requirements of individual species.

Tinctures

Alcohol has been used to make herbal extracts for millennia, with evidence coming from as far back as 6000 BCE. Chemical analysis of clay-pot residues found in China from this era revealed a fermented beverage made with grapes, honey and hawthorn berries. Evidence exists of wines, beers and other fermented herbal beverages being produced and consumed for medicinal purposes as far back as 3000 BCE in Egypt and 2000 BCE in the Americas.

Tinctures are made by soaking ("macerating") an herb in an alcohol-water mixture (the "menstruum") over a period of time. This encourages the active plant constituents to dissolve, giving tinctures a relatively stronger action than herbal infusions or decoctions.

There are three main advantages of using alcohol:

1. It is the only edible solvent that will successfully extract and preserve a very high percentage of the naturally occurring herbal constituents that are otherwise poorly soluble in water.
2. It is a great natural preservative (ethanol concentrations above 30 per cent by volume work best to maximize the shelf life of the extracts).
3. It is an excellent carrying agent that facilitates the herbal constituents' absorption into the bloodstream.

The simplest form of tincturing is known as maceration and can be carried out by using either of the two following methods.

Dry Herb Tincture

This is probably the most common way of tincturing plant material. The dried herb, either finely chopped, ground or powdered, is soaked in an ethanol-water mixture for a minimum of two weeks. A standard dry herb tincture is generally made using a weight (dried herb material) to volume (alcohol and water) ratio of 1:5 (e.g., 1 gram of dried herb material to 5 millilitres of ethanol-water mix). An ethanol-water mix of 40 to 60 per cent ethanol by volume is used, depending on the herb, part of the plant and constituents that are being extracted.

Initially, stir the mixture well, making sure that all of the herb is wet and ideally covered by a quarter inch of menstruum. Keep the maceration in a dark place, giving it a shake daily, and then, after a minimum of 14 days, pour it through a muslin cloth or such like, and press out the herbs (or "marc"), removing as much extract as possible.

Sometimes it is essential to dry down an herb before tincturing, as drying can increase the active ingredient desired or break down potential toxins present in the fresh plant material.

For each dry herb being tinctured, it's advisable to consult a reference work such as a materia medica or a pharmacopoeia, which will give specifics on the weight to volume ratio and the percentage strength of ethanol to be used.

Fresh Herb Tincture

When tincturing fresh plant material, using a higher-strength alcohol (95 per cent) is beneficial, as dilution will naturally occur because of the significant water content of the fresh plants or roots.

One part (by weight) of the fresh, chopped herb is soaked (macerated) in two parts (by volume) of 190 proof or 95 per cent alcohol (a 1:2 ratio). There is no need to blend or shake this maceration: the tincture is formed passively as a result of dehydration, the ethanol rupturing the plant cell walls and drawing plant constituents and water into the solution, leaving only cellulose and dead tissue behind. The maceration is steeped for at least 14 days and then, as with the dry herb tincture method, strained and the marc pressed out.

Tinctures produced by both maceration techniques are best stored in coloured glass or in the dark, to protect them from degradation by light, and at a constant, relatively cool temperature, if possible.

A single dose of tincture may vary from a few drops to a teaspoon or tablespoon, depending on the herb and its constituents. Again, consulting a materia medica or pharmacopoeia is important for determining the dose of each herb, as some are what are known as "low-dose botanicals," and too much tincture can be extremely unpleasant or, in a few very rare instances, fatal.

The amount of alcohol in a single tincture dose is quite small. If desired, some of the alcohol may be evaporated off by adding the tincture dose to half a cup of hot water: stir, let it sit for a minute and then take. Some active herbal constituents can be damaged by hot or boiling water, so, again, consulting various herbal sources can be helpful.

Many herbalists feel that, through sense and biochemical stimulation, aroma and taste are an important part of the medicinal action of the tincture. For optimal results, add the tincture dose to 2 to 4 ounces of warm water, then sip and savour the flavour and aroma; although you may not always like the taste, allow the herb to begin the healing process that is Plant Medicine.

Medicinal Perennials to Know and Grow... and Know Even More

An Afterword by Dan Jason

Maybe the above should have been the title of this book. It is one thing to read about herbs, another to start growing them and still another to truly experience them.

Rupert Adams and I have been growing and using the plants in this book for many years. And we are still getting to know them.

It is remarkable that, even with little or no historical contact, cultures around the world have valued and honoured similar tried-and-true benefits of these medicinals. As well, many of these herbs have a depth of healing possibilities, resulting in different but effective uses in different cultures.

Unlike pharmaceutical drugs, these medicines don't carry so many contraindications that it becomes scary to think of using them. The fact that it is you who is choosing the herb makes a huge difference. You wouldn't imbibe an energizing plant like Maral Root if you wanted a good night's sleep, and you wouldn't brew a nervine such as Hops if you wanted to be energized.

In fact, these herbs present themselves in a totally different manner than prescription drugs. They speak to the potential of self-care rather than dictated care. They open channels of self-empowerment and self-awareness. It's not a difficult stretch to regulate dosage and frequency of these herbs for whatever condition you have or don't have. It's as simple as learning not to have coffee after 2 in the afternoon, or not to have more than two cups a day, or not to have any at all.

These herbs are indeed "big time," having been tested for thousands of years. But that doesn't mean you shouldn't test them yourself in a careful and responsible manner. At first, take small amounts of tea or tincture to observe its effects on you. Most of them are aids to healthy balance and immunity, rather than a silver bullet that will annihilate your unwanted state of mind or body.

Over the years, I have learned subtle differences between similar-acting medicinals. For example, I have found Skullcap, Hops and Valerian to be wonderful nervines that are conducive to restful sleep; now I know intuitively which one will work best when my agitated mind is reluctant to slow down.

For Rupert and me, the smells of the flower or root and the taste of the tincture or tea are an important part of the healing energy of these plants—not to mention the beauty of their flowers and foliage, plus the birds, bees and butterflies they attract! The years fly by, and these amazing plants keep offering us their blessings, just as they have since humans first started embracing them.

More than 50 years ago, I wrote a bestselling book with some friends called *Some Useful Wild Plants*. In it, I attested that the deepest healing comes through knowledge and self-realization. These plants can be powerful allies in that process. Just as good gardening comes from good observation, good healing comes from paying attention to the garden that is your body.

During my years with Salt Spring Seeds, a company that sells simple, saveable, organically grown seeds, it has been heartwarming to see the veritable explosion in the number of people wanting to grow their own food. Considering the state of the world these days, that hasn't surprised me. What I didn't anticipate is the fact that Salt Spring Seeds' medicinal herb seeds have been outselling all our other seed categories!

In terms of self-care, these medicinals offer us the ability to take care not only of ourselves but also of each other. Historically, these medicinal herbs have never been much about money, but about community. They are almost anti-money and pro-community by their very nature. They keep being there for us. Each plant offers countless seeds each year and can also be multiplied by cuttings or divisions. As medicine goes, there aren't too many things easier than drying some leaves or making a tincture that has a very long shelf life.

So perhaps the full title for this book should have been: *Medicinal Perennials to Know and Grow... and Know Even More... and Share!*

Here's hoping these herbs give you and your community much healing and health, beauty and joy.

References

A tremendous amount of information about all the medicinal perennials in this book is now available on the internet. We have done a lot of research there ourselves and have been surprised to find so many excellent sources for starting, growing and processing these herbs into medicine. There are even many videos by enthusiastic growers that make techniques for cultivation and usage easily grasped. As well, you'll discover page after page of citations of scientific experiments, including many very recent ones that have been done to confirm traditional uses of these plants and / or to reveal new ones.

If you want to find out more about these medicinals, we encourage you to do some Google searching. We have found it best to look for the plant as well as to type in the aspects of the herb that interest you the most. You'll notice that very different entries appear depending on whether you are looking for growing, processing, historical or medical information. As with everything these days, information can vary depending on outlook and approach, but generally we believe you'll find basic agreement with everything we've written in this book. We urge you to read as many posts as you reasonably can and come to your own conclusions about how to grow and use these herbs, as well as about their healing power and safety.

We have both been passionate herbalists for many decades, starting long before you could source information with just a click or two. Most of our learning has come from actual experience, oral communications and books. Below are some of the most inspiring and comprehensive books we know.

Andrew Chevallier, *Encyclopedia of Herbal Medicine: 550 Herbs and Remedies for Common Ailments* (DK, 2016).

David Hoffmann, *Medical Herbalism: The Science and Practice of Herbal Medicine* (Healing Arts Press, 2003).

Margaret Grieve, *A Modern Herbal* (Stone Basin Books, 2015).

Matthew Wood, *The Book of Herbal Wisdom: Using Plants as Medicines* (North Atlantic Books, 1997).

Michael Moore, *Medicinal Plants of the Pacific West* (Museum of New Mexico Press, 2011).

Michael Tierra, *The Way of Herbs* (Pocket Books, 1998).

Peg Schafer, *The Chinese Medicinal Herb Farm: A Cultivator's Guide to Small-Scale Organic Herb Production* (Chelsea Green Publishing, 2011).

Steven Foster, *Herbal Renaissance: Growing, Using and Understanding Herbs in the Modern World* (Gibbs Smith, 1993).

Terry Breverton, *Breverton's Complete Herbal: A Book of Remarkable Plants and Their Uses* (Lyons Press, 2012).

About the Authors and Artist

Lyn Alice

Born creative, Lyn Alice studied at the American Academy of Art in Chicago and at the Denver Botanic Gardens School of Botanical Art & Illustration. She did extensive studies in Rome, Florence and Venice. Her passion for illustration developed through years of experience in the commercial and fine arts. Striving to create beauty in all she does, her work reflects an expressive painterly approach in lifestyle and botanical illustration. This is her second book with Dan Jason and Salt Spring Seeds; *Changing the Climate with the Seeds We Sow* is still a bestseller. She loves collaborating with others in the industry. She lives in southern Georgia with her dog and horse, Obi and Moses. "My Life is Art!" Her diverse portfolio can be seen at lynalice.com, and you can order fine art prints of the illustrations in this book. Her email is mail@lynalice.com.

Rupert Adams

Rupert Adams is an award-winning brewmaster; social and environmental activist; retired music-events promoter, booking agent and DJ; yoga teacher; and medicinal herb, food and seed grower. He has worked for nearly two decades with Dan Jason, currently growing a wide variety of vegetable, grain and herb seeds for Salt Spring Seeds and the BC Eco Seed Co-op. He specializes in growing medicinal herbs, running his own medicinal herb and tincture business, Kairos Botanicals. Rupert worked for three years as a coordinator and advisor with the Bauta Family Initiative on Canadian Seed Security. He currently resides and grows at Abundance Community Farm in Agassiz, BC.

Dan Jason

Dan Jason has owned and operated the mail-order seed company Salt Spring Seeds since 1986 (saltspringseeds.com). He is the author of over a dozen books on organic gardening and agriculture, including *Some Useful Wild Plants* and *Saving Seeds: A Home Gardener's Guide to Preserving Plant Biodiversity*. Dan and his wife, Celeste, live at Seed Spirit Farm on Salt Spring Island, BC. Dan's email is dan@saltspringseeds.com.